Chapter 1: The Foundation of Memory and Homeostasis: An Introduction to the Hippocampus and Hypothalamus

Introduction

Nestled deep within the human brain, two structures, the hippocampus and the hypothalamus, play pivotal roles in shaping our cognitive abilities and physiological functions. These interconnected regions, part of the limbic system, are responsible for memory formation, spatial navigation, stress responses, and the regulation of essential bodily functions. This chapter will provide a comprehensive overview of these two structures, exploring their anatomical, physiological, and functional characteristics.

The Hippocampus: The Memory Maker

The hippocampus, derived from the Greek word for "seahorse" due to its distinctive shape, is a key player in memory formation and retrieval. Located within the temporal lobe, it is primarily responsible for converting short-term memories into long-term memories. This process, known as memory consolidation, involves the strengthening of neural connections in the hippocampus and other brain regions.

Anatomical Structure and Connections

The hippocampus consists of several distinct regions, including the dentate gyrus, Ammon's horn (CA1-CA4), and the subiculum. These regions are interconnected through a complex network of neural pathways, forming the hippocampal circuit. The hippocampus receives input from various cortical areas, including the entorhinal cortex, which serves as a gateway for information from the neocortex.

Memory Formation and Retrieval

The hippocampus is crucial for the formation of declarative memories, which include both semantic (factual) and episodic (personal experiences) memories. During memory formation, incoming information is processed by the hippocampus, where it is encoded and stored as a neural representation. This process involves the strengthening of synaptic connections between neurons through long-term potentiation (LTP), a cellular mechanism that underlies learning and memory.

Retrieving memories involves reactivating the neural networks that were involved in their initial encoding. The hippocampus plays a key role in guiding this retrieval process, working in conjunction with other brain regions to access and recall stored information.

The Hypothalamus: The Master Regulator

The hypothalamus, a small but powerful brain region located below the thalamus, serves as the body's master regulator. It plays a critical role in maintaining homeostasis, the body's internal balance, by controlling a wide range of physiological functions, including hunger, thirst, body temperature, sleep-wake cycles, and stress responses.

Anatomical Structure and Connections

The hypothalamus is composed of numerous nuclei, each with specific functions. These nuclei are interconnected and receive input from various brain regions, including the hippocampus, amygdala, and cerebral cortex. The hypothalamus also has extensive connections with the pituitary gland, a key endocrine organ that regulates hormone secretion.

Homeostasis and Physiological Regulation

The hypothalamus plays a central role in maintaining energy balance by regulating hunger and satiety. It contains specialized neurons that sense changes in blood glucose levels and hormone concentrations, triggering appropriate responses to maintain adequate energy intake. The hypothalamus also regulates thirst by monitoring fluid balance and stimulating the release of antidiuretic hormone (ADH) to conserve water.

In addition to energy balance, the hypothalamus controls body temperature by coordinating responses such as shivering, sweating, and changes in blood flow. It also regulates sleep-wake cycles by interacting with the suprachiasmatic nucleus (SCN), the body's internal clock.

The Hippocampus and Hypothalamus: A Dynamic Duo

While the hippocampus and hypothalamus have distinct functions, they are closely interconnected and interact in complex ways. The hippocampus plays a role in regulating stress responses by influencing the hypothalamic-pituitary-adrenal (HPA) axis, a key neuroendocrine pathway involved in stress. The hypothalamus, in turn, can influence hippocampal function by modulating neurotransmitter levels and synaptic plasticity.

The hippocampus and hypothalamus also interact in the context of spatial navigation. The hippocampus is involved in creating cognitive maps of the environment, while the hypothalamus plays a role in regulating locomotor activity and orienting behavior.

Conclusion

The hippocampus and hypothalamus are two essential brain regions that play critical roles in memory, homeostasis, and behavior. These structures are interconnected and interact in complex ways to regulate a wide range of physiological functions. A deeper understanding of the hippocampus and hypothalamus is crucial for developing effective treatments for neurodegenerative diseases, psychiatric disorders, and metabolic disorders.

Chapter 2: Anatomy and Physiology of the Hippocampus

Introduction

The hippocampus, a small, seahorse-shaped structure located within the temporal lobe, plays a crucial role in memory formation and retrieval. Its intricate anatomical structure and complex physiological processes underlie its cognitive functions. This chapter will provide a detailed exploration of the hippocampus's anatomy and physiology, including its distinct regions, neural pathways, and cellular mechanisms.

Anatomical Structure

The hippocampus is composed of several interconnected regions, each with specific functions. These regions include:

- **Dentate gyrus:** A thin, convoluted layer of gray matter that receives input from the entorhinal cortex.
- **Cornu Ammonis (CA) regions:** These regions are further divided into CA1, CA2, and CA3. CA1 is particularly vulnerable to damage in conditions such as Alzheimer's disease, while CA3 plays a critical role in pattern completion.
- **Subiculum:** A transitional area that connects the hippocampus to the entorhinal cortex.

The hippocampus is part of the limbic system, a network of brain regions involved in emotion, memory, and motivation. It has extensive connections with other brain areas, including the prefrontal cortex, amygdala, and hypothalamus.

Neural Pathways

The hippocampus is characterized by its unique circuitry, known as the hippocampal circuit. This circuit involves a series of interconnected regions that work together to process and store information. The primary pathway within the hippocampal circuit is the trisynaptic pathway, which begins in the entorhinal cortex and passes through the dentate gyrus, CA3, and CA1 regions before returning to the entorhinal cortex.

Cellular Mechanisms

The hippocampus is composed of a diverse array of neurons, including pyramidal cells, granule cells, and interneurons. These neurons communicate with each other through synapses, where neurotransmitters are released to transmit signals. The hippocampus is particularly rich in glutamate receptors, which play a crucial role in synaptic plasticity, the ability of synapses to change their strength in response to experience.

One of the most important cellular mechanisms underlying hippocampal function is long-term potentiation (LTP). LTP is a persistent increase in synaptic strength that occurs when a synapse is repeatedly stimulated. It is believed to be a key mechanism for memory formation and consolidation.

The Role of the Hippocampus in Memory Formation

The hippocampus is essential for the consolidation of short-term memories into long-term memories. This process involves the strengthening of synaptic connections between neurons in the hippocampus and other brain regions. The trisynaptic pathway plays a particularly important role in this process, as it allows for the repeated activation of neurons and the strengthening of their connections.

The hippocampus is also involved in the retrieval of stored memories. When we try to recall a memory, the hippocampus helps to reactivate the neural networks that were involved in its encoding. This process involves the coordinated activity of multiple regions within the hippocampus and the retrieval of information from other brain areas.

Conclusion

The hippocampus is a complex brain structure with a unique anatomy and physiology. Its interconnected regions, neural pathways, and cellular mechanisms underlie its critical role in memory formation and retrieval. A deeper understanding of the hippocampus is essential for developing effective treatments for memory disorders and other neurological conditions.

Chapter 3: Memory Consolidation and Retrieval: The Hippocampus's Critical Role

Introduction

The hippocampus, a small, seahorse-shaped structure within the temporal lobe, plays a pivotal role in transforming short-term memories into long-term memories. This process, known as memory consolidation, is essential for retaining information and experiences over time. In this chapter, we will explore the intricate mechanisms involved in memory consolidation and retrieval, focusing on the hippocampus's critical role in these processes.

Memory Consolidation: From Short-Term to Long-Term

Memory consolidation is a complex process that involves the transfer of information from short-term memory, a temporary storage system with limited capacity, to long-term memory, a more permanent storage system with virtually unlimited capacity. The hippocampus is a key player in this process, acting as a bridge between these two memory systems.

The Role of the Hippocampus

The hippocampus is believed to be involved in the initial encoding and consolidation of new memories. During this process, incoming information is processed by the hippocampus, where it is transformed into a neural representation. This representation is then strengthened through a process known as long-term potentiation (LTP), which involves the strengthening of synaptic connections between neurons.

The Systems Consolidation Theory

One prominent theory of memory consolidation is the systems consolidation theory, which posits that the hippocampus is initially involved in the consolidation of new memories, but over time, these memories are gradually transferred to other brain regions, such as the neocortex. This transfer process is thought to be mediated by the hippocampus, which acts as a temporary storage site for new memories until they are consolidated in the neocortex.

The Role of Sleep

Sleep plays a crucial role in memory consolidation. During sleep, the hippocampus replays memories, allowing for their strengthening and integration into long-term memory. This process is thought to be mediated by the interaction between the hippocampus and the neocortex, which occurs during slow-wave sleep.

Memory Retrieval: Accessing Stored Memories

The hippocampus is also involved in the retrieval of stored memories. When we try to recall a memory, the hippocampus helps to reactivate the neural networks that were involved in its encoding. This process involves the coordinated activity of multiple brain regions, including the prefrontal cortex, which is involved in attention and decision-making.

The Role of Cues

Cues can help us to retrieve memories more easily. Cues can be internal, such as emotional states or physical sensations, or external, such as locations or objects. The hippocampus is thought to play a role in associating memories with cues, making it easier to retrieve them when the appropriate cue is present.

The Impact of Aging and Disease

Aging and certain neurological diseases, such as Alzheimer's disease, can impair memory consolidation and retrieval. In these conditions, the hippocampus may be damaged, leading to difficulties in forming and retrieving new memories.

Conclusion

The hippocampus is a critical brain region for memory consolidation and retrieval. Its role in transforming short-term memories into long-term memories and retrieving stored information is essential for our ability to learn, remember, and adapt to our environment. A deeper understanding of the hippocampus's role in memory processes can inform the development of treatments for memory disorders and other cognitive impairments.

Chapter 4: Spatial Navigation and Place Cells: The Hippocampus's Cognitive Map

Introduction

The hippocampus, a small, seahorse-shaped structure within the temporal lobe, plays a crucial role in spatial navigation. It acts as a cognitive map, allowing us to represent and navigate our environment. In this chapter, we will explore the hippocampus's role in spatial navigation, focusing on the concept of place cells and their importance in understanding how we represent and navigate our surroundings.

Place Cells: A Neural Representation of Space

Place cells are neurons located in the hippocampus that fire when an animal is in a specific location within its environment. These cells create a neural representation of space, allowing us to mentally map out our surroundings and navigate efficiently.

Discovery of Place Cells

The discovery of place cells by John O'Keefe and his colleagues in the 1970s revolutionized our understanding of the hippocampus's role in spatial navigation. O'Keefe and his team recorded the activity of hippocampal neurons in rats as they explored a novel environment. They found that many of these neurons fired selectively in specific locations within the environment, indicating that they were encoding the animal's position.

Properties of Place Cells

Place cells exhibit several key properties:

- **Place-specific firing:** Place cells fire selectively in a specific location within the environment, creating a neural representation of that location.
- **Remapping:** Place cells can remap their firing fields when the environment is changed. This allows us to adapt our spatial representation to new environments.
- **Phase precession:** Place cells exhibit phase precession, which means that their firing rate increases as the animal approaches their preferred location within the environment.

The Hippocampal Circuit and Spatial Navigation

The hippocampus is part of a larger network of brain regions involved in spatial navigation. The entorhinal cortex, which provides input to the hippocampus, is also involved in spatial representation. The hippocampus and entorhinal cortex work together to create and maintain a cognitive map of the environment.

Grid Cells

Grid cells are neurons located in the entorhinal cortex that fire in a hexagonal grid pattern. These cells provide a framework for spatial representation, allowing us to orient ourselves within our environment. Grid cells interact with place cells to create a more precise spatial representation.

The Role of the Hippocampus in Spatial Memory

The hippocampus is also involved in spatial memory, the ability to remember the location of objects and places. Place cells play a crucial role in spatial memory by encoding the location of objects and landmarks within the environment. The hippocampus also helps us to navigate back to previously visited locations by reactivating the neural networks associated with those locations.

The Hippocampus and Disease

Impairments in spatial navigation and memory are common symptoms of neurological disorders, such as Alzheimer's disease and Parkinson's disease. These impairments are often associated with damage to the hippocampus. Understanding the hippocampus's role in spatial navigation and memory can inform the development of treatments for these conditions.

Conclusion

The hippocampus plays a critical role in spatial navigation and memory. Place cells, which fire selectively in specific locations within the environment, create a neural representation of space. The hippocampus and entorhinal cortex work together to create and maintain a cognitive map of the environment. A deeper understanding of the hippocampus's role in spatial navigation can inform the development of treatments for neurological disorders that affect spatial memory.

Chapter 5: The Hippocampus in Learning and Plasticity

Introduction

The hippocampus, a small, seahorse-shaped structure within the temporal lobe, plays a crucial role in learning and memory. Its unique anatomical structure and physiological properties allow it to adapt to new experiences and form lasting memories. In this chapter, we will explore the hippocampus's role in learning and plasticity, focusing on its involvement in various learning paradigms and the underlying cellular mechanisms.

The Hippocampus as a Learning Machine

The hippocampus is a highly plastic brain region, meaning that it can change its structure and function in response to experience. This plasticity is essential for learning and memory, as it allows the hippocampus to form new neural connections and strengthen existing ones.

Classical Conditioning

The hippocampus is involved in classical conditioning, a type of learning in which an organism associates a neutral stimulus with a meaningful stimulus. For example, in Pavlov's famous experiment, dogs learned to associate the sound of a bell with the presentation of food. The hippocampus is thought to play a role in forming the association between the neutral stimulus and the meaningful stimulus.

Operant Conditioning

The hippocampus is also involved in operant conditioning, a type of learning in which an organism's behavior is modified by its consequences. For example, a rat may learn to press a lever to obtain a reward. The hippocampus is thought to play a role in forming the association between the behavior and the reward.

Declarative Memory

The hippocampus is particularly important for declarative memory, which includes both semantic (factual) and episodic (personal experiences) memories. The hippocampus is involved in the encoding, consolidation, and retrieval of declarative memories.

Cellular Mechanisms of Learning and Plasticity

The hippocampus's ability to learn and form memories is based on its unique cellular properties. One of the most important mechanisms underlying learning and plasticity in the hippocampus is long-term potentiation (LTP). LTP is a persistent increase in synaptic strength that occurs when a synapse is repeatedly stimulated. It is believed to be a key mechanism for memory formation and consolidation.

Synaptic Plasticity

Synaptic plasticity is the ability of synapses to change their strength in response to experience. LTP is one type of synaptic plasticity, but there are also other forms, such as long-term depression (LTD). LTD is a decrease in synaptic strength that occurs when a synapse is repeatedly stimulated at a low frequency.

Neurotransmitters

Neurotransmitters play a crucial role in synaptic plasticity. Glutamate is a particularly important neurotransmitter in the hippocampus, as it is involved in LTP and LTD. Other neurotransmitters, such as dopamine and acetylcholine, also play a role in learning and plasticity.

The Hippocampus and Disease

Impairments in learning and memory are common symptoms of neurological disorders, such as Alzheimer's disease and Parkinson's disease. These impairments are often associated with damage to the hippocampus. Understanding the hippocampus's role in learning and plasticity can inform the development of treatments for these conditions.

Conclusion

The hippocampus is a highly plastic brain region that plays a crucial role in learning and memory. Its unique cellular properties allow it to form new neural connections and strengthen existing ones, enabling us to acquire new knowledge and skills. A deeper understanding of the hippocampus's role in learning and plasticity can inform the development of treatments for cognitive impairments and other neurological disorders.

Chapter 6: The Hippocampus and Disease

Introduction

The hippocampus, a small, seahorse-shaped structure within the temporal lobe, plays a critical role in memory formation and retrieval. However, when the hippocampus is damaged or impaired, it can lead to a variety of cognitive and neurological disorders. In this chapter, we will explore the relationship between the hippocampus and disease, focusing on neurodegenerative diseases, mood disorders, and other conditions that affect hippocampal function.

Neurodegenerative Diseases

Neurodegenerative diseases, such as Alzheimer's disease and Parkinson's disease, are characterized by the progressive loss of neurons. The hippocampus is particularly vulnerable to damage in these diseases, leading to significant memory impairments.

Alzheimer's Disease

Alzheimer's disease is the most common cause of dementia. It is characterized by the formation of amyloid plaques and neurofibrillary tangles, which damage neurons in the hippocampus and other brain regions. The loss of hippocampal neurons contributes to memory loss, disorientation, and other cognitive symptoms of Alzheimer's disease.

Parkinson's Disease

Parkinson's disease is a neurodegenerative disorder characterized by the loss of dopamine-producing neurons in the substantia nigra. While Parkinson's disease is primarily associated with motor symptoms, it can also affect cognitive function, including memory and attention. The hippocampus may be involved in the cognitive symptoms of Parkinson's disease.

Mood Disorders

Mood disorders, such as depression and anxiety, are common mental health conditions that can affect hippocampal function. Studies have shown that individuals with depression often have reduced hippocampal volume and altered hippocampal function.

Depression

Depression is a complex disorder with a variety of causes. The hippocampus plays a role in the regulation of mood, and damage to the hippocampus may contribute to depressive symptoms. Stress, which can negatively impact hippocampal function, is also a risk factor for depression.

Anxiety

Anxiety is a common mental health condition characterized by excessive worry and fear. The hippocampus is involved in fear conditioning, a type of learning that associates a neutral stimulus with a negative outcome. Dysfunctional hippocampal function may contribute to anxiety disorders.

Other Hippocampal Disorders

In addition to neurodegenerative diseases and mood disorders, the hippocampus can be affected by other conditions, including:

- **Schizophrenia:** Studies have shown that individuals with schizophrenia often have reduced hippocampal volume and altered hippocampal function.
- **Epilepsy:** The hippocampus is a common site of seizure activity in patients with temporal lobe epilepsy.
- **Post-traumatic stress disorder (PTSD):** Stress can negatively impact hippocampal function, and PTSD is a condition that is often associated with exposure to traumatic events.

Therapeutic Interventions

A variety of therapeutic interventions can be used to target hippocampal dysfunction. These include:

- **Pharmacological treatments:** Medications can be used to treat neurodegenerative diseases, mood disorders, and other conditions that affect hippocampal function.
- **Cognitive-behavioral therapy:** This type of therapy can help individuals with depression and anxiety to manage their symptoms and improve their quality of life.
- **Deep brain stimulation:** This technique involves implanting electrodes into the brain to stimulate specific regions. It has been shown to be effective in treating Parkinson's disease and depression.

Conclusion

The hippocampus is a vulnerable brain region that can be affected by a variety of diseases. Understanding the relationship between the hippocampus and disease is essential for developing effective treatments and improving the quality of life for individuals with these conditions.

Chapter 7: Anatomy and Physiology of the Hypothalamus

Introduction

The hypothalamus, a small but powerful brain region located below the thalamus, plays a critical role in regulating a wide range of physiological functions. It acts as the body's master regulator, controlling everything from hunger and thirst to body temperature and stress responses. In this chapter, we will explore the anatomy and physiology of the hypothalamus, including its distinct nuclei, neural pathways, and hormonal functions.

Anatomical Structure

The hypothalamus is a complex structure composed of numerous nuclei, each with specific functions. These nuclei can be grouped into three major divisions:

- **Anterior hypothalamus:** This region is involved in regulating body temperature, thirst, and appetite.
- **Lateral hypothalamus:** This region is involved in regulating hunger, thirst, and arousal.
- **Posterior hypothalamus:** This region is involved in regulating body temperature, sleep-wake cycles, and stress responses.

The hypothalamus is also connected to the pituitary gland, a crucial endocrine organ that secretes hormones into the bloodstream. The hypothalamus controls the pituitary gland through both neural and hormonal signals.

Neural Pathways

The hypothalamus is interconnected with many other brain regions, including the hippocampus, amygdala, and cerebral cortex. These connections allow the hypothalamus to receive and integrate information from various sources, allowing it to regulate physiological functions effectively.

One of the most important neural pathways involving the hypothalamus is the hypothalamic-pituitary-adrenal (HPA) axis. This axis plays a crucial role in the stress response, and it involves the hypothalamus, the pituitary gland, and the adrenal glands.

Hormonal Functions

The hypothalamus plays a critical role in regulating the release of hormones from the pituitary gland. These hormones include:

- **Growth hormone:** This hormone is important for growth, development, and metabolism.
- **Thyroid-stimulating hormone (TSH):** This hormone stimulates the thyroid gland to produce thyroid hormones, which regulate metabolism.
- **Adrenocorticotropic hormone (ACTH):** This hormone stimulates the adrenal glands to produce cortisol, a stress hormone.
- **Luteinizing hormone (LH) and follicle-stimulating hormone (FSH):** These hormones regulate reproductive function.
- **Prolactin:** This hormone stimulates milk production in breastfeeding women.

The hypothalamus also produces its own hormones, such as oxytocin and vasopressin. Oxytocin is involved in social bonding, childbirth, and milk production, while vasopressin is involved in water balance and blood pressure regulation.

Conclusion

The hypothalamus is a complex brain region that plays a crucial role in regulating a wide range of physiological functions. Its anatomical structure, neural pathways, and hormonal functions allow it to act as the body's master regulator. A deeper understanding of the hypothalamus is essential for understanding the underlying mechanisms of various diseases and disorders.

Chapter 8: Homeostasis and Energy Balance: The Hypothalamus's Role

Introduction

The hypothalamus, a small but powerful brain region located below the thalamus, plays a critical role in maintaining homeostasis, the body's internal balance. One of the most important aspects of homeostasis is energy balance, which involves regulating hunger, thirst, and metabolism. In this chapter, we will explore the hypothalamus's role in energy balance and its involvement in obesity and other metabolic disorders.

The Hypothalamus and Hunger

The hypothalamus contains several nuclei that are involved in regulating hunger. The lateral hypothalamus, in particular, is known as the "feeding center" because it stimulates hunger when activated. The arcuate nucleus, located within the hypothalamus, contains neurons that produce neuropeptides such as neuropeptide Y (NPY) and agouti-related protein (AgRP). These neuropeptides stimulate hunger by activating pathways in the brain that promote food intake.

The Hypothalamus and Satiety

The hypothalamus also contains nuclei that are involved in regulating satiety, the feeling of fullness after a meal. The ventromedial hypothalamus (VMH) is known as the "satiety center" because it inhibits hunger when activated. The arcuate nucleus also contains neurons that produce proopiomelanocortin (POMC) and cocaine-amphetamine-regulated transcript (CART). These neuropeptides inhibit hunger by activating pathways in the brain that reduce food intake.

The Role of Hormones

Hormones play a crucial role in regulating hunger and satiety. The hormones leptin and ghrelin are particularly important. Leptin is produced by adipose tissue and is a signal of energy stores. When leptin levels are high, it signals the brain to reduce hunger. Ghrelin is produced by the stomach and is a signal of hunger. When ghrelin levels are high, it stimulates the brain to increase hunger.

The Hypothalamus and Obesity

Obesity is a complex disorder that is characterized by excessive body fat. The hypothalamus plays a role in regulating energy balance, and disruptions in hypothalamic function can contribute to obesity. For example, individuals with obesity may have resistance to leptin, a hormone that signals satiety. This can lead to increased hunger and decreased energy expenditure.

The Hypothalamus and Diabetes

The hypothalamus is also involved in regulating glucose metabolism. Disruptions in hypothalamic function can contribute to type 2 diabetes, a condition characterized by insulin resistance and hyperglycemia. The hypothalamus plays a role in regulating the release of insulin and glucagon, hormones that control blood sugar levels.

Therapeutic Interventions

A variety of therapeutic interventions can be used to target hypothalamic dysfunction and treat obesity and other metabolic disorders. These interventions include:

- **Lifestyle modifications:** Changes in diet and exercise can help to improve energy balance and reduce the risk of obesity and diabetes.
- **Pharmacological treatments:** Medications can be used to target the hypothalamus and regulate hunger, satiety, and metabolism.
- **Surgical interventions:** In some cases, surgical procedures may be used to treat obesity by reducing the size of the stomach or bypassing parts of the digestive system.

Conclusion

The hypothalamus plays a critical role in regulating energy balance and homeostasis. Disruptions in hypothalamic function can contribute to obesity, diabetes, and other metabolic disorders. A deeper understanding of the hypothalamus's role in energy balance can inform the development of effective treatments for these conditions.

Chapter 9: Stress Response and the Hypothalamic-Pituitary-Adrenal (HPA) Axis

Introduction

The hypothalamus, a small but powerful brain region located below the thalamus, plays a critical role in regulating the body's stress response. This response is mediated by the hypothalamic-pituitary-adrenal (HPA) axis, a complex neuroendocrine system that involves the hypothalamus, the pituitary gland, and the adrenal glands. In this chapter, we will explore the HPA axis and its role in the stress response, as well as the impact of chronic stress on the hypothalamus and its functions.

The HPA Axis: A Stress Response System

The HPA axis is a complex network of interconnected structures that work together to regulate the body's response to stress. When faced with a stressor, the hypothalamus releases corticotropin-releasing hormone (CRH), which stimulates the pituitary gland to release adrenocorticotropic hormone (ACTH). ACTH, in turn, stimulates the adrenal glands to produce cortisol, a stress hormone.

Cortisol has a variety of effects on the body, including:

- **Mobilizing energy:** Cortisol increases blood sugar levels and mobilizes fat stores for energy.
- **Suppressing the immune system:** Cortisol can suppress the immune system to conserve energy.
- **Influencing mood and cognition:** Cortisol can affect mood and cognitive function, particularly memory and attention.

The Role of the Hypothalamus in the HPA Axis

The hypothalamus plays a central role in regulating the HPA axis. It receives information from various brain regions, including the amygdala and hippocampus, about the presence of a stressor. The hypothalamus then integrates this information and determines the appropriate level of stress response.

The hypothalamus can also regulate the HPA axis through negative feedback. When cortisol levels become too high, they can signal the hypothalamus to reduce CRH release, which in turn reduces ACTH and cortisol production.

Chronic Stress and the Hypothalamus

Chronic stress can have a negative impact on the hypothalamus and its functions. Prolonged exposure to stress can lead to:

- **Hypercortisolism:** Excessive cortisol production can lead to a variety of health problems, including obesity, high blood pressure, and diabetes.
- **Hippocampal atrophy:** Chronic stress can cause the hippocampus to shrink, which can impair memory and learning.
- **Dysregulation of the HPA axis:** Chronic stress can disrupt the normal functioning of the HPA axis, leading to a variety of problems.

The Impact of Stress on the Hippocampus

The hippocampus is particularly vulnerable to the effects of chronic stress. Stress can cause the hippocampus to shrink and lose neurons, which can impair memory and learning. This may be due to the increased levels of cortisol, which can damage hippocampal neurons.

Therapeutic Interventions

A variety of therapeutic interventions can be used to target the HPA axis and reduce the negative effects of chronic stress. These interventions include:

- **Stress management techniques:** Mindfulness meditation, yoga, and exercise can help to reduce stress levels.
- **Pharmacological treatments:** Medications can be used to reduce cortisol levels and improve the functioning of the HPA axis.
- **Psychotherapy:** Psychotherapy can help individuals to cope with stress and develop healthy coping mechanisms.

Conclusion

The hypothalamus plays a critical role in regulating the stress response through the HPA axis. Chronic stress can have a negative impact on the hypothalamus and its functions, leading to a variety of health problems. Understanding the role of the hypothalamus in the stress response can inform the development of effective treatments for stress-related disorders.

Chapter 10: Sleep-Wake Cycles and Circadian Rhythms: The Hypothalamus's Role

Introduction

The hypothalamus, a small but powerful brain region located below the thalamus, plays a critical role in regulating sleep-wake cycles and circadian rhythms. These biological rhythms are essential for maintaining optimal health and well-being. In this chapter, we will explore the hypothalamus's role in sleep-wake regulation, the circadian clock, and the impact of sleep disorders on the hypothalamus.

The Hypothalamus and Sleep-Wake Regulation

The hypothalamus contains several nuclei that are involved in regulating sleep-wake cycles. The suprachiasmatic nucleus (SCN), located within the hypothalamus, is the body's primary circadian clock. The SCN receives input from the retina, which detects light and dark signals from the environment. This information helps the SCN to synchronize the body's internal clock with the external environment.

The hypothalamus also interacts with other brain regions involved in sleep-wake regulation, such as the brainstem and thalamus. These regions help to regulate the transition between sleep and wakefulness, as well as the different stages of sleep.

The Circadian Clock

The circadian clock is a biological rhythm that regulates various physiological functions, including sleep-wake cycles, hormone secretion, and body temperature. The SCN is the primary location of the circadian clock in mammals. The SCN contains a network of neurons that oscillate in a 24-hour cycle, allowing the body to anticipate daily changes in light and dark.

The circadian clock is influenced by a variety of factors, including light, temperature, and social cues. Disruptions to the circadian clock can lead to sleep disorders and other health problems.

Sleep Disorders and the Hypothalamus

Sleep disorders can have a significant impact on health and well-being. The hypothalamus plays a role in regulating sleep-wake cycles, and disruptions in hypothalamic function can contribute to sleep disorders.

Insomnia

Insomnia is a common sleep disorder characterized by difficulty falling asleep or staying asleep. The hypothalamus may be involved in regulating sleep-wake cycles, and disruptions in hypothalamic function can contribute to insomnia.

Narcolepsy

Narcolepsy is a sleep disorder characterized by excessive daytime sleepiness and sudden sleep attacks. The hypothalamus contains neurons that produce orexin, a neurotransmitter that regulates wakefulness. Narcolepsy is often caused by a deficiency in orexin.

Sleep apnea

Sleep apnea is a sleep disorder characterized by pauses in breathing during sleep. The hypothalamus plays a role in regulating breathing, and disruptions in hypothalamic function can contribute to sleep apnea.

Therapeutic Interventions

A variety of therapeutic interventions can be used to treat sleep disorders and improve sleep quality. These interventions include:

- **Lifestyle changes:** Changes in sleep habits, diet, and exercise can help to improve sleep quality.
- **Pharmacological treatments:** Medications can be used to treat insomnia, narcolepsy, and sleep apnea.
- **Cognitive-behavioral therapy:** This type of therapy can help individuals with insomnia to develop healthy sleep habits.

Conclusion

The hypothalamus plays a critical role in regulating sleep-wake cycles and circadian rhythms. Disruptions in hypothalamic function can contribute to sleep disorders, which can have a significant impact on health and well-being. Understanding the hypothalamus's role in sleep regulation can inform the development of effective treatments for sleep disorders.

Chapter 11: Reproductive Behavior and Hormones: The Hypothalamus's Role

Introduction

The hypothalamus, a small but powerful brain region located below the thalamus, plays a critical role in regulating reproductive behavior and hormone secretion. It acts as a central hub for integrating information from various sources, including the brain, endocrine system, and environment, to coordinate reproductive functions. In this chapter, we will explore the hypothalamus's role in reproductive behavior and hormone regulation, as well as its involvement in reproductive disorders.

The Hypothalamus and Reproductive Hormones

The hypothalamus plays a crucial role in regulating the secretion of reproductive hormones from the pituitary gland. These hormones include:

- **Gonadotropin-releasing hormone (GnRH):** GnRH stimulates the pituitary gland to release luteinizing hormone (LH) and follicle-stimulating hormone (FSH). LH and FSH are essential for the development and function of the reproductive organs.
-
- **Oxytocin:** Oxytocin is a hormone that is involved in childbirth, milk production, and social bonding.
- **Vasopressin:** Vasopressin is a hormone that is involved in water balance and blood pressure regulation. It also plays a role in social behavior and pair bonding.

The hypothalamus receives input from various sources, including the brain, endocrine system, and environment. This information helps the hypothalamus to regulate the secretion of reproductive hormones in response to changing conditions.

The Hypothalamus and Reproductive Behavior

The hypothalamus also plays a role in regulating reproductive behavior, including mating, pregnancy, and parenting. The hypothalamus contains neurons that produce and release neurotransmitters, such as dopamine and serotonin, that are involved in regulating sexual behavior. The hypothalamus also interacts with other brain regions, such as the amygdala and prefrontal cortex, to coordinate reproductive behavior.

The Hypothalamus and Reproductive Disorders

Disruptions in hypothalamic function can lead to a variety of reproductive disorders, including:

- **Infertility:** Difficulty conceiving can be caused by a variety of factors, including hypothalamic dysfunction.
- **Premature menopause:** Premature menopause is the cessation of menstruation before the age of 40. It can be caused by hypothalamic dysfunction.
- **Sexual dysfunction:** Sexual dysfunction can be caused by a variety of factors, including hypothalamic dysfunction.

Therapeutic Interventions

A variety of therapeutic interventions can be used to treat reproductive disorders and improve reproductive function. These interventions include:

- **Hormone therapy:** Hormone therapy can be used to replace missing hormones and improve reproductive function.
- **Surgery:** In some cases, surgery may be necessary to treat reproductive disorders, such as endometriosis or polycystic ovary syndrome.
- **Lifestyle changes:** Changes in diet, exercise, and stress management can help to improve reproductive health.

Conclusion

The hypothalamus plays a critical role in regulating reproductive behavior and hormone secretion. Disruptions in hypothalamic function can lead to a variety of reproductive disorders. A deeper understanding of the hypothalamus's role in reproduction can inform the development of effective treatments for these disorders.

Chapter 12: The Hippocampus-Hypothalamus Circuit: A Dynamic Duo

Introduction

The hippocampus and hypothalamus, two key structures within the limbic system, are intimately interconnected and work together to regulate a wide range of physiological and cognitive functions. This chapter will explore the intricate relationship between the hippocampus and hypothalamus, examining their anatomical connections, functional interactions, and the implications for behavior and disease.

Anatomical Connections

The hippocampus and hypothalamus are connected through a complex network of neural pathways. The fornix, a prominent white matter tract, directly connects the hippocampus to the hypothalamus. Additionally, the hippocampus receives input from the hypothalamus through the mammillary bodies, a pair of nuclei located in the hypothalamus. These connections facilitate bidirectional communication between the two structures, allowing for the integration of information and coordination of responses.

Functional Interactions: Memory and Stress

The hippocampus and hypothalamus play critical roles in memory formation and stress responses, respectively. Their interaction is particularly important in the context of stress-related memory. The hippocampus is involved in encoding and consolidating memories, while the hypothalamus regulates the body's stress response through the hypothalamic-pituitary-adrenal (HPA) axis.

- **Stress-Induced Memory Impairment:** Chronic stress can impair hippocampal function, leading to difficulties in memory formation and retrieval. This is partly due to the elevated cortisol levels associated with stress, which can damage hippocampal neurons.
- **The Role of the Hypothalamus:** The hypothalamus plays a role in modulating the hippocampus's response to stress. It can influence the release of neurotransmitters that affect hippocampal function, such as norepinephrine and dopamine.

Functional Interactions: Homeostasis and Behavior

The hippocampus and hypothalamus also interact in regulating homeostasis and behavior. The hypothalamus is involved in maintaining the body's internal balance, while the hippocampus plays a role in spatial navigation and decision-making.

- **Spatial Navigation and Stress:** The hippocampus is essential for spatial navigation, and stress can impair hippocampal function. The hypothalamus may play a role in mediating the effects of stress on spatial navigation.
- **Homeostasis and Behavior:** The hippocampus and hypothalamus interact in regulating various aspects of behavior, including feeding, drinking, and sexual behavior. The hypothalamus plays a central role in regulating these behaviors, while the hippocampus may provide contextual information and influence decision-making.

Implications for Disease

The hippocampus and hypothalamus are often implicated in various neurological and psychiatric disorders. Dysfunctional interactions between these two structures can contribute to:

- **Neurodegenerative Diseases:** Alzheimer's disease and Parkinson's disease are associated with damage to the hippocampus and hypothalamus.
- **Mood Disorders:** Depression and anxiety are often linked to alterations in hippocampal and hypothalamic function.
- **Substance Abuse:** The hippocampus and hypothalamus play roles in reward processing and addiction, and their interactions may contribute to substance abuse disorders.

Therapeutic Implications

Understanding the interactions between the hippocampus and hypothalamus can inform the development of therapeutic interventions for various disorders. For example, targeting the hippocampus and hypothalamus may be beneficial for treating memory impairments, mood disorders, and substance abuse.

Conclusion

The hippocampus and hypothalamus form a dynamic duo, working together to regulate a wide range of physiological and cognitive functions. Their intricate anatomical connections and functional interactions are essential for maintaining normal behavior and preventing disease. Future research on the hippocampus-hypothalamus circuit will continue to shed light on the underlying mechanisms of brain function and inform the development of new therapeutic strategies.

Chapter 13: Memory and Stress: The Hippocampus-Hypothalamus Connection

Introduction

The hippocampus and hypothalamus, two key structures within the limbic system, play critical roles in memory formation and stress responses, respectively. Their intricate interplay is particularly evident in the context of stress-related memory impairments. This chapter will delve into the complex relationship between memory and stress, exploring how the hippocampus and hypothalamus interact to mediate these processes.

The Hippocampus and Memory

The hippocampus is a vital brain region for declarative memory, which encompasses both semantic (factual) and episodic (personal experiences) memories. Its role in memory formation and retrieval is well-established, involving processes such as encoding, consolidation, and retrieval.

- **Encoding:** The hippocampus receives sensory information, processes it, and transforms it into a neural representation that can be stored.
- **Consolidation:** Over time, these newly formed memories are strengthened and stabilized through a process known as consolidation, often facilitated during sleep.
- **Retrieval:** When needed, the hippocampus helps to reactivate these stored memories, allowing us to recall past events.

The Hypothalamus and Stress

The hypothalamus, acting as a central regulator, orchestrates the body's response to stress through the hypothalamic-pituitary-adrenal (HPA) axis. This axis involves the release of cortisol, a stress hormone, which has widespread effects on the body, including:

- **Energy mobilization:** Cortisol increases blood sugar levels and mobilizes fat stores for energy.
- **Immune system suppression:** Cortisol can temporarily suppress the immune system to conserve resources.
- **Influencing mood and cognition:** Cortisol can affect mood and cognitive functions, including memory.

The Hippocampus-Hypothalamus Interaction in Stress

The hippocampus and hypothalamus are interconnected, and their interactions are particularly relevant in the context of stress. Chronic stress can lead to:

- **Hippocampal Atrophy:** Excessive cortisol levels associated with chronic stress can lead to the shrinkage of the hippocampus, a phenomenon known as hippocampal atrophy.
- **Impaired Memory:** This atrophy can result in difficulties with memory formation and retrieval, particularly for emotionally charged events.
- **Feedback Loop:** The hippocampus can also influence the HPA axis. It plays a role in regulating the release of cortisol, potentially acting as a negative feedback mechanism to prevent excessive stress responses.

Stress-Related Memory Impairments

The interaction between the hippocampus and hypothalamus can lead to various stress-related memory impairments, including:

- **Post-Traumatic Stress Disorder (PTSD):** Individuals with PTSD often exhibit difficulties in memory consolidation and retrieval, particularly for traumatic memories.
- **Depression:** Depression can be associated with memory deficits, and the hippocampus is thought to play a role in these impairments.
- **Exam Anxiety:** Stress experienced during exams can interfere with memory retrieval, leading to poorer performance.

Therapeutic Implications

Understanding the hippocampus-hypothalamus connection in stress-related memory impairments can inform the development of therapeutic interventions. Strategies targeting both the hippocampus and hypothalamus may be beneficial, such as:

- **Stress Reduction Techniques:** Mindfulness meditation, yoga, and exercise can help reduce stress levels and protect the hippocampus from damage.
- **Pharmacological Interventions:** Medications that modulate cortisol levels or target hippocampal function may be helpful in treating stress-related memory impairments.
- **Cognitive-Behavioral Therapy:** This type of therapy can help individuals manage stress and improve their coping mechanisms.

Conclusion

The hippocampus and hypothalamus form a dynamic duo in regulating memory and stress. Their intricate interactions are crucial for understanding the impact of stress on cognitive function. By exploring the mechanisms underlying stress-related memory impairments, researchers can develop more effective therapeutic strategies to help individuals cope with the challenges posed by chronic stress.

Chapter 14: The Hippocampus and Homeostasis: A Dynamic Duo

Introduction

The hippocampus and hypothalamus, two key structures within the limbic system, play critical roles in memory formation and homeostasis, respectively. While their functions may seem distinct, these two regions are interconnected and collaborate to regulate various aspects of behavior and physiology. This chapter will explore the dynamic relationship between the hippocampus and hypothalamus, focusing on their roles in energy balance, appetite control, and metabolic processes.

The Hypothalamus and Homeostasis

The hypothalamus, often referred to as the body's "master regulator," is responsible for maintaining homeostasis, the body's internal balance. This includes regulating essential physiological functions such as body temperature, hunger, thirst, and metabolism.

- **Energy Balance:** The hypothalamus plays a crucial role in regulating energy balance, ensuring that the body has enough energy to meet its needs. It contains specialized neurons that sense changes in blood glucose levels and hormone concentrations, triggering appropriate responses to maintain adequate energy intake and expenditure.
- **Appetite Control:** The hypothalamus houses the "feeding center" and "satiety center," which regulate hunger and fullness. These regions receive signals from various hormones and neurotransmitters, helping to determine when to eat and how much to consume.
- **Metabolic Processes:** The hypothalamus also influences metabolic processes, such as the rate at which the body burns calories. It interacts with other endocrine glands, such as the thyroid and adrenal glands, to regulate metabolism and ensure that the body has enough energy for its needs.

The Hippocampus and Homeostasis

While the hippocampus is primarily associated with memory formation and retrieval, it also plays a role in regulating certain aspects of homeostasis. Recent studies have highlighted the hippocampus's involvement in:

- **Energy Regulation:** The hippocampus may influence the hypothalamus's control of energy balance, potentially by providing contextual information about the environment and the body's needs.
- **Stress-Related Eating:** Stress can affect eating behavior, and the hippocampus plays a role in regulating the stress response. Dysfunctional hippocampal activity may contribute to stress-induced eating, leading to weight gain and metabolic imbalances.
- **Circadian Rhythms:** The hippocampus interacts with the hypothalamus to regulate circadian rhythms, which influence sleep-wake cycles and metabolic processes. Disruptions in circadian rhythms can affect energy balance and contribute to obesity and other metabolic disorders.

The Hippocampus–Hypothalamus Circuit in Obesity and Metabolic Disorders

Dysfunctional interactions between the hippocampus and hypothalamus have been implicated in obesity and metabolic disorders. For example, studies have shown that individuals with obesity may have altered hippocampal structure and function, potentially affecting their ability to regulate energy balance and appetite. Additionally, stress-induced changes in the hippocampus and hypothalamus may contribute to weight gain and metabolic imbalances.

Therapeutic Implications

Understanding the hippocampus-hypothalamus circuit in the context of energy balance and metabolic disorders can inform the development of therapeutic interventions. Targeting these regions may be beneficial for treating obesity, diabetes, and other metabolic conditions. For example, strategies aimed at improving hippocampal function or reducing stress levels may help to regulate energy balance and prevent weight gain.

Conclusion

The hippocampus and hypothalamus, while often studied separately, are interconnected and collaborate to regulate various aspects of homeostasis, including energy balance, appetite control, and metabolic processes. Dysfunctional interactions between these regions can contribute to obesity, diabetes, and other metabolic disorders. Future research on the hippocampus-hypothalamus circuit will provide valuable insights into the underlying mechanisms of these conditions and inform the development of effective therapeutic strategies.

Chapter 15: Future Directions and Emerging Research

Introduction

The hippocampus and hypothalamus, two key structures within the limbic system, continue to be the subject of intense research. Advances in neuroscience technology and methodologies have opened up new avenues for exploring the complex interactions between these regions and their roles in various cognitive and physiological functions. This chapter will delve into the exciting field of emerging research, highlighting potential future directions and the implications for understanding the brain and developing novel therapeutic strategies.

Neuroimaging Techniques

- **Advanced MRI Techniques:** Diffusion tensor imaging (DTI) and functional MRI (fMRI) have provided invaluable insights into the structural and functional connectivity of the hippocampus and hypothalamus. Future advancements in these techniques may allow for even more precise mapping and analysis of neural networks.
- **Optogenetics:** This revolutionary technique enables researchers to control the activity of specific neurons using light. Optogenetics can be used to study the causal relationships between hippocampal and hypothalamic activity and behavior.
- **In Vivo Electrophysiology:** Techniques such as single-unit recording and calcium imaging allow for the precise measurement of neuronal activity in real time, providing valuable information about the neural circuits underlying hippocampal and hypothalamic functions.

Molecular and Cellular Biology

- **Epigenetics:** Epigenetic modifications, such as DNA methylation and histone acetylation, can alter gene expression and influence brain function. Research is exploring the role of epigenetics in regulating hippocampal and hypothalamic development and plasticity.
- **Neurogenesis:** The hippocampus is known for its neurogenesis, the process of generating new neurons. Understanding the factors that regulate neurogenesis may provide insights into potential therapeutic strategies for brain disorders.
- **Neurotransmitters and Receptors:** Advances in understanding the role of neurotransmitters and receptors in hippocampal and hypothalamic function are ongoing. Identifying novel targets for therapeutic intervention may lead to the development of more effective treatments.

Computational Neuroscience

- **Neural Networks:** Computational models of the hippocampus and hypothalamus are being developed to simulate their complex interactions and predict their behavior. These models can help to test hypotheses and generate new insights.
- **Machine Learning:** Machine learning algorithms can be used to analyze large datasets of neural activity and identify patterns that may be relevant to hippocampal and hypothalamic function.

Therapeutic Implications

- **Personalized Medicine:** Advances in neuroscience may enable the development of personalized treatments based on an individual's unique genetic makeup and brain function.
- **Brain-Computer Interfaces:** Brain-computer interfaces (BCIs) may be used to restore lost functions or enhance cognitive abilities in individuals with brain disorders or injuries.
- **Neuroprosthetic Devices:** Neuroprosthetic devices can be implanted into the brain to stimulate specific regions and improve function. These devices may be used to treat conditions such as depression, anxiety, and memory disorders.

Ethical Considerations

- **Privacy and Consent:** As neuroscience research advances, it is essential to address ethical concerns related to data privacy and informed consent.
- **Dual-Use Concerns:** The potential for misuse of neuroscience technology, such as in developing mind-control weapons, raises ethical questions.

Conclusion

The field of neuroscience is rapidly evolving, and the hippocampus and hypothalamus remain at the forefront of research. Future advancements in technology and methodologies will undoubtedly lead to new discoveries and insights into the complex interactions between these brain regions and their roles in behavior and disease. By addressing ethical concerns and harnessing the potential of emerging technologies, researchers can continue to make significant contributions to our understanding of the brain and develop innovative therapeutic strategies.

Chapter 16: Future Directions and Emerging Research

Introduction

The hippocampus and hypothalamus, two key structures within the limbic system, continue to be the subject of intense research. Advances in neuroscience technology and methodologies have opened up new avenues for exploring the complex interactions between these regions and their roles in various cognitive and physiological functions. This chapter will delve into the exciting field of emerging research, highlighting potential future directions and the implications for understanding the brain and developing novel therapeutic strategies.

Neuroimaging Techniques

- **Advanced MRI Techniques:** Diffusion tensor imaging (DTI) and functional MRI (fMRI) have provided invaluable insights into the structural and functional connectivity of the hippocampus and hypothalamus. Future advancements in these techniques may allow for even more precise mapping and analysis of neural networks.
- **Optogenetics:** This revolutionary technique enables researchers to control the activity of specific neurons using light. Optogenetics can be used to study the causal relationships between hippocampal and hypothalamic activity and behavior.
- **In Vivo Electrophysiology:** Techniques such as single-unit recording and calcium imaging allow for the precise measurement of neuronal activity in real time, providing valuable information about the neural circuits underlying hippocampal and hypothalamic functions.

Molecular and Cellular Biology

- **Epigenetics:** Epigenetic modifications, such as DNA methylation and histone acetylation, can alter gene expression and influence brain function. Research is exploring the role of epigenetics in regulating hippocampal and hypothalamic development and plasticity.
- **Neurogenesis:** The hippocampus is known for its neurogenesis, the process of generating new neurons. Understanding the factors that regulate neurogenesis may provide insights into potential therapeutic strategies for brain disorders.
- **Neurotransmitters and Receptors:** Advances in understanding the role of neurotransmitters and receptors in hippocampal and hypothalamic function are ongoing. Identifying novel targets for therapeutic intervention may lead to the development of more effective treatments.

Computational Neuroscience

- **Neural Networks:** Computational models of the hippocampus and hypothalamus are being developed to simulate their complex interactions and predict their behavior. These models can help to test hypotheses and generate new insights.
- **Machine Learning:** Machine learning algorithms can be used to analyze large datasets of neural activity and identify patterns that may be relevant to hippocampal and hypothalamic function.

Therapeutic Implications

- **Personalized Medicine:** Advances in neuroscience may enable the development of personalized treatments based on an individual's unique genetic makeup and brain function.
- **Brain-Computer Interfaces:** Brain-computer interfaces (BCIs) may be used to restore lost functions or enhance cognitive abilities in individuals with brain disorders or injuries.
- **Neuroprosthetic Devices:** Neuroprosthetic devices can be implanted into the brain to stimulate specific regions and improve function. These devices may be used to treat conditions such as depression, anxiety, and memory disorders.

Ethical Considerations

- **Privacy and Consent:** As neuroscience research advances, it is essential to address ethical concerns related to data privacy and informed consent.
- **Dual-Use Concerns:** The potential for misuse of neuroscience technology, such as in developing mind-control weapons, raises ethical questions.

Conclusion

The field of neuroscience is rapidly evolving, and the hippocampus and hypothalamus remain at the forefront of research. Future advancements in technology and methodologies will undoubtedly lead to new discoveries and insights into the complex interactions between these brain regions and their roles in behavior and disease. By addressing ethical concerns and harnessing the potential of emerging technologies, researchers can continue to make significant contributions to our understanding of the brain and develop innovative therapeutic strategies.

Chapter 17: Emerging Therapeutic Strategies for Hippocampal and Hypothalamic Dysfunction

Introduction

The hippocampus and hypothalamus, two critical brain regions involved in memory, emotion, and homeostasis, are implicated in a variety of neurological and psychiatric disorders. As our understanding of these structures and their functions continues to evolve, so too do the therapeutic strategies being developed to address associated conditions. This chapter will explore some of the most promising emerging therapeutic approaches targeting hippocampal and hypothalamic dysfunction.

Pharmacological Interventions

- **Neuroprotective Agents:** Research is focused on identifying compounds that can protect hippocampal and hypothalamic neurons from damage. This includes exploring the potential of antioxidants, anti-inflammatory agents, and neurotrophic factors.
- **Modulation of Neurotransmitters:** Targeting neurotransmitters involved in hippocampal and hypothalamic function, such as glutamate, GABA, dopamine, and serotonin, holds promise for treating disorders like depression, anxiety, and memory impairments.
- **Hormone Therapies:** Manipulating hormonal pathways, particularly the hypothalamic-pituitary-adrenal (HPA) axis, is being investigated for conditions like stress-related disorders and metabolic disturbances.

Non-Pharmacological Interventions

- **Brain-Computer Interfaces (BCIs):** BCIs aim to restore lost functions or enhance cognitive abilities by establishing communication between the brain and external devices. They may be particularly useful for treating memory impairments or motor deficits associated with hippocampal and hypothalamic dysfunction.
- **Deep Brain Stimulation (DBS):** This technique involves implanting electrodes into specific brain regions to deliver electrical stimulation. DBS has shown promise in treating conditions like depression, obsessive-compulsive disorder, and Parkinson's disease, which often involve hippocampal and hypothalamic dysfunction.
- **Transcranial Magnetic Stimulation (TMS):** TMS uses magnetic fields to stimulate specific areas of the brain. It has been explored as a potential treatment for depression, anxiety, and memory impairments.
- **Cognitive-Behavioral Therapy (CBT):** CBT can help individuals develop coping strategies for stress, anxiety, and depression, which can indirectly impact hippocampal and hypothalamic function.

Stem Cell Therapies

- **Neural Stem Cell Transplantation:** The transplantation of neural stem cells into the brain has shown potential for repairing damaged tissue and promoting neurogenesis in animal models. Clinical trials are exploring the feasibility of this approach for treating neurodegenerative diseases like Alzheimer's and Parkinson's.
- **Induced Pluripotent Stem Cells (iPSCs):** iPSCs can be generated from adult cells and then differentiated into various cell types, including neurons. This technology offers a promising avenue for studying hippocampal and hypothalamic function and developing personalized therapies.

Lifestyle Interventions

- **Exercise:** Regular physical activity has been shown to have beneficial effects on brain health, including improving cognitive function and reducing stress.
- **Diet:** A healthy diet rich in nutrients can support brain health and reduce the risk of neurodegenerative diseases.
- **Stress Management:** Techniques such as mindfulness meditation, yoga, and deep breathing can help manage stress and reduce its negative impact on the hippocampus and hypothalamus.

Personalized Medicine

- **Genetic Testing:** Identifying genetic factors that contribute to hippocampal and hypothalamic dysfunction can help to tailor treatments to individual patients.
- **Precision Medicine:** By combining genetic information with clinical data and neuroimaging techniques, researchers can develop more personalized and effective therapeutic strategies.

Ethical Considerations

- **Consent and Safety:** Ensuring informed consent and minimizing risks associated with emerging therapeutic strategies is crucial.
- **Equity and Access:** Efforts should be made to ensure that new treatments are accessible to all patients, regardless of socioeconomic status or geographic location.

Conclusion

The field of hippocampal and hypothalamic research is rapidly evolving, and emerging therapeutic strategies hold great promise for improving the lives of individuals with brain disorders. By combining innovative technologies, personalized medicine, and lifestyle interventions, researchers can develop more effective and targeted treatments for conditions such as memory impairments, mood disorders, and neurodegenerative diseases.

Chapter 18: Future Directions and Emerging Research

Introduction

The hippocampus and hypothalamus, two key structures within the limbic system, continue to be the subject of intense research. Advances in neuroscience technology and methodologies have opened up new avenues for exploring the complex interactions between these regions and their roles in various cognitive and physiological functions. This chapter will delve into the exciting field of emerging research, highlighting potential future directions and the implications for understanding the brain and developing novel therapeutic strategies.

Neuroimaging Techniques

- **Advanced MRI Techniques:** Diffusion tensor imaging (DTI) and functional MRI (fMRI) have provided invaluable insights into the structural and functional connectivity of the hippocampus and hypothalamus. Future advancements in these techniques may allow for even more precise mapping and analysis of neural networks.
- **Optogenetics:** This revolutionary technique enables researchers to control the activity of specific neurons using light. Optogenetics can be used to study the causal relationships between hippocampal and hypothalamic activity and behavior.
- **In Vivo Electrophysiology:** Techniques such as single-unit recording and calcium imaging allow for the precise measurement of neuronal activity in real time, providing valuable information about the neural circuits underlying hippocampal and hypothalamic functions.

Molecular and Cellular Biology

- **Epigenetics:** Epigenetic modifications, such as DNA methylation and histone acetylation, can alter gene expression and influence brain function. Research is exploring the role of epigenetics in regulating hippocampal and hypothalamic development and plasticity.
- **Neurogenesis:** The hippocampus is known for its neurogenesis, the process of generating new neurons. Understanding the factors that regulate neurogenesis may provide insights into potential therapeutic strategies for brain disorders.
- **Neurotransmitters and Receptors:** Advances in understanding the role of neurotransmitters and receptors in hippocampal and hypothalamic function are ongoing. Identifying novel targets for therapeutic intervention may lead to the development of more effective treatments.

Computational Neuroscience

- **Neural Networks:** Computational models of the hippocampus and hypothalamus are being developed to simulate their complex interactions and predict their behavior. These models can help to test hypotheses and generate new insights.
- **Machine Learning:** Machine learning algorithms can be used to analyze large datasets of neural activity and identify patterns that may be relevant to hippocampal and hypothalamic function.

Therapeutic Implications

- **Personalized Medicine:** Advances in neuroscience may enable the development of personalized treatments based on an individual's unique genetic makeup and brain function.
- **Brain-Computer Interfaces:** Brain-computer interfaces (BCIs) may be used to restore lost functions or enhance cognitive abilities in individuals with brain disorders or injuries.
- **Neuroprosthetic Devices:** Neuroprosthetic devices can be implanted into the brain to stimulate specific regions and improve function. These devices may be used to treat conditions such as depression, anxiety, and memory disorders.

Ethical Considerations

- **Privacy and Consent:** As neuroscience research advances, it is essential to address ethical concerns related to data privacy and informed consent.
- **Dual-Use Concerns:** The potential for misuse of neuroscience technology, such as in developing mind-control weapons, raises ethical questions.

Conclusion

The field of neuroscience is rapidly evolving, and the hippocampus and hypothalamus remain at the forefront of research. Future advancements in technology and methodologies will undoubtedly lead to new discoveries and insights into the complex interactions between these brain regions and their roles in behavior and disease. By addressing ethical concerns and harnessing the potential of emerging technologies, researchers can continue to make significant contributions to our understanding of the brain and develop innovative therapeutic strategies.

Chapter 19: Future Directions and Emerging Research

Introduction

The hippocampus and hypothalamus, two key structures within the limbic system, continue to be the subject of intense research. Advances in neuroscience technology and methodologies have opened up new avenues for exploring the complex interactions between these regions and their roles in various cognitive and physiological functions. This chapter will delve into the exciting field of emerging research, highlighting potential future directions and the implications for understanding the brain and developing novel therapeutic strategies.

Neuroimaging Techniques

- **Advanced MRI Techniques:** Diffusion tensor imaging (DTI) and functional MRI (fMRI) have provided invaluable insights into the structural and functional connectivity of the hippocampus and hypothalamus. Future advancements in these techniques may allow for even more precise mapping and analysis of neural networks.
- **Optogenetics:** This revolutionary technique enables researchers to control the activity of specific neurons using light. Optogenetics can be used to study the causal relationships between hippocampal and hypothalamic activity and behavior.
- **In Vivo Electrophysiology:** Techniques such as single-unit recording and calcium imaging allow for the precise measurement of neuronal activity in real time, providing valuable information about the neural circuits underlying hippocampal and hypothalamic functions.

Molecular and Cellular Biology

- **Epigenetics:** Epigenetic modifications, such as DNA methylation and histone acetylation, can alter gene expression and influence brain function. Research is exploring the role of epigenetics in regulating hippocampal and hypothalamic development and plasticity.
- **Neurogenesis:** The hippocampus is known for its neurogenesis, the process of generating new neurons. Understanding the factors that regulate neurogenesis may provide insights into potential therapeutic strategies for brain disorders.
- **Neurotransmitters and Receptors:** Advances in understanding the role of neurotransmitters and receptors in hippocampal and hypothalamic function are ongoing. Identifying novel targets for therapeutic intervention may lead to the development of more effective treatments.

Computational Neuroscience

- **Neural Networks:** Computational models of the hippocampus and hypothalamus are being developed to simulate their complex interactions and predict their behavior. These models can help to test hypotheses and generate new insights.
- **Machine Learning:** Machine learning algorithms can be used to analyze large datasets of neural activity and identify patterns that may be relevant to hippocampal and hypothalamic function.

Therapeutic Implications

- **Personalized Medicine:** Advances in neuroscience may enable the development of personalized treatments based on an individual's unique genetic makeup and brain function.
- **Brain-Computer Interfaces:** Brain-computer interfaces (BCIs) may be used to restore lost functions or enhance cognitive abilities in individuals with brain disorders or injuries.
- **Neuroprosthetic Devices:** Neuroprosthetic devices can be implanted into the brain to stimulate specific regions and improve function. These devices may be used to treat conditions such as depression, anxiety, and memory disorders.

Ethical Considerations

- **Privacy and Consent:** As neuroscience research advances, it is essential to address ethical concerns related to data privacy and informed consent.
- **Dual-Use Concerns:** The potential for misuse of neuroscience technology, such as in developing mind-control weapons, raises ethical questions.

Conclusion

The field of neuroscience is rapidly evolving, and the hippocampus and hypothalamus remain at the forefront of research. Future advancements in technology and methodologies will undoubtedly lead to new discoveries and insights into the complex interactions between these brain regions and their roles in behavior and disease. By addressing ethical concerns and harnessing the potential of emerging technologies, researchers can continue to make significant contributions to our understanding of the brain and develop innovative therapeutic strategies.

Chapter 20: Future Directions and Emerging Research

Introduction

The hippocampus and hypothalamus, two key structures within the limbic system, continue to be the subject of intense research. Advances in neuroscience technology and methodologies have opened up new avenues for exploring the complex interactions between these regions and their roles in various cognitive and physiological functions. This chapter will delve into the exciting field of emerging research, highlighting potential future directions and the implications for understanding the brain and developing novel therapeutic strategies.

Neuroimaging Techniques

- **Advanced MRI Techniques:** Diffusion tensor imaging (DTI) and functional MRI (fMRI) have provided invaluable insights into the structural and functional connectivity of the hippocampus and hypothalamus. Future advancements in these techniques may allow for even more precise mapping and analysis of neural networks.
- **Optogenetics:** This revolutionary technique enables researchers to control the activity of specific neurons using light. Optogenetics can be used to study the causal relationships between hippocampal and hypothalamic activity and behavior.
- **In Vivo Electrophysiology:** Techniques such as single-unit recording and calcium imaging allow for the precise measurement of neuronal activity in real time, providing valuable information about the neural circuits underlying hippocampal and hypothalamic functions.

Molecular and Cellular Biology

- **Epigenetics:** Epigenetic modifications, such as DNA methylation and histone acetylation, can alter gene expression and influence brain function. Research is exploring the role of epigenetics in regulating hippocampal and hypothalamic development and plasticity.
- **Neurogenesis:** The hippocampus is known for its neurogenesis, the process of generating new neurons. Understanding the factors that regulate neurogenesis may provide insights into potential therapeutic strategies for brain disorders.
- **Neurotransmitters and Receptors:** Advances in understanding the role of neurotransmitters and receptors in hippocampal and hypothalamic function are ongoing. Identifying novel targets for therapeutic intervention may lead to the development of more effective treatments.

Computational Neuroscience

- **Neural Networks:** Computational models of the hippocampus and hypothalamus are being developed to simulate their complex interactions and predict their behavior. These models can help to test hypotheses and generate new insights.
- **Machine Learning:** Machine learning algorithms can be used to analyze large datasets of neural activity and identify patterns that may be relevant to hippocampal and hypothalamic function.

Therapeutic Implications

- **Personalized Medicine:** Advances in neuroscience may enable the development of personalized treatments based on an individual's unique genetic makeup and brain function.
- **Brain-Computer Interfaces:** Brain-computer interfaces (BCIs) may be used to restore lost functions or enhance cognitive abilities in individuals with brain disorders or injuries.
- **Neuroprosthetic Devices:** Neuroprosthetic devices can be implanted into the brain to stimulate specific regions and improve function. These devices may be used to treat conditions such as depression, anxiety, and memory disorders.

Ethical Considerations

- **Privacy and Consent:** As neuroscience research advances, it is essential to address ethical concerns related to data privacy and informed consent.
- **Dual-Use Concerns:** The potential for misuse of neuroscience technology, such as in developing mind-control weapons, raises ethical questions.

Conclusion

The field of neuroscience is rapidly evolving, and the hippocampus and hypothalamus remain at the forefront of research. Future advancements in technology and methodologies will undoubtedly lead to new discoveries and insights into the complex interactions between these brain regions and their roles in behavior and disease. By addressing ethical concerns and harnessing the potential of emerging technologies, researchers can continue to make significant contributions to our understanding of the brain and develop innovative therapeutic strategies.

Chapter 21: Future Directions and Emerging Research

Introduction

The hippocampus and hypothalamus, two key structures within the limbic system, continue to be the subject of intense research. Advances in neuroscience technology and methodologies have opened up new avenues for exploring the complex interactions between these regions and their roles in various cognitive and physiological functions. This chapter will delve into the exciting field of emerging research, highlighting potential future directions and the implications for understanding the brain and developing novel therapeutic strategies.

Neuroimaging Techniques

- **Advanced MRI Techniques:** Diffusion tensor imaging (DTI) and functional MRI (fMRI) have provided invaluable insights into the structural and functional connectivity of the hippocampus and hypothalamus. Future advancements in these techniques may allow for even more precise mapping and analysis of neural networks.
- **Optogenetics:** This revolutionary technique enables researchers to control the activity of specific neurons using light. Optogenetics can be used to study the causal relationships between hippocampal and hypothalamic activity and behavior.
- **In Vivo Electrophysiology:** Techniques such as single-unit recording and calcium imaging allow for the precise measurement of neuronal activity in real time, providing valuable information about the neural circuits underlying hippocampal and hypothalamic functions.

Molecular and Cellular Biology

- **Epigenetics:** Epigenetic modifications, such as DNA methylation and histone acetylation, can alter gene expression and influence brain function. Research is exploring the role of epigenetics in regulating hippocampal and hypothalamic development and plasticity.
- **Neurogenesis:** The hippocampus is known for its neurogenesis, the process of generating new neurons. Understanding the factors that regulate neurogenesis may provide insights into potential therapeutic strategies for brain disorders.
- **Neurotransmitters and Receptors:** Advances in understanding the role of neurotransmitters and receptors in hippocampal and hypothalamic function are ongoing. Identifying novel targets for therapeutic intervention may lead to the development of more effective treatments.

Computational Neuroscience

- **Neural Networks:** Computational models of the hippocampus and hypothalamus are being developed to simulate their complex interactions and predict their behavior. These models can help to test hypotheses and generate new insights.
- **Machine Learning:** Machine learning algorithms can be used to analyze large datasets of neural activity and identify patterns that may be relevant to hippocampal and hypothalamic function.

Therapeutic Implications

- **Personalized Medicine:** Advances in neuroscience may enable the development of personalized treatments based on an individual's unique genetic makeup and brain function.
- **Brain-Computer Interfaces:** Brain-computer interfaces (BCIs) may be used to restore lost functions or enhance cognitive abilities in individuals with brain disorders or injuries.
- **Neuroprosthetic Devices:** Neuroprosthetic devices can be implanted into the brain to stimulate specific regions and improve function. These devices may be used to treat conditions such as depression, anxiety, and memory disorders.

Ethical Considerations

- **Privacy and Consent:** As neuroscience research advances, it is essential to address ethical concerns related to data privacy and informed consent.
- **Dual-Use Concerns:** The potential for misuse of neuroscience technology, such as in developing mind-control weapons, raises ethical questions.

Conclusion

The field of neuroscience is rapidly evolving, and the hippocampus and hypothalamus remain at the forefront of research. Future advancements in technology and methodologies will undoubtedly lead to new discoveries and insights into the complex interactions between these brain regions and their roles in behavior and disease. By addressing ethical concerns and harnessing the potential of emerging technologies, researchers can continue to make significant contributions to our understanding of the brain and develop innovative therapeutic strategies.

Chapter 22: Emerging Therapeutic Strategies for Hippocampal and Hypothalamic Dysfunction

Introduction

The hippocampus and hypothalamus, two critical brain regions involved in memory, emotion, and homeostasis, are implicated in a variety of neurological and psychiatric disorders. As our understanding of these structures and their functions continues to evolve, so too do the therapeutic strategies being developed to address associated conditions. This chapter will explore some of the most promising emerging therapeutic approaches targeting hippocampal and hypothalamic dysfunction.

Pharmacological Interventions

- **Neuroprotective Agents:** Research is focused on identifying compounds that can protect hippocampal and hypothalamic neurons from damage. This includes exploring the potential of antioxidants, anti-inflammatory agents, and neurotrophic factors.
- **Modulation of Neurotransmitters:** Targeting neurotransmitters involved in hippocampal and hypothalamic function, such as glutamate, GABA, dopamine, and serotonin, holds promise for treating disorders like depression, anxiety, and memory impairments.
- **Hormone Therapies:** Manipulating hormonal pathways, particularly the hypothalamic-pituitary-adrenal (HPA) axis, is being investigated for conditions like stress-related disorders and metabolic disturbances.

Non-Pharmacological Interventions

- **Brain-Computer Interfaces (BCIs):** BCIs aim to restore lost functions or enhance cognitive abilities by establishing communication between the brain and external devices. They may be particularly useful for treating memory impairments or motor deficits associated with hippocampal and hypothalamic dysfunction.
- **Deep Brain Stimulation (DBS):** This technique involves implanting electrodes into specific brain regions to deliver electrical stimulation. DBS has shown promise in treating conditions like depression, obsessive-compulsive disorder, and Parkinson's disease, which often involve hippocampal and hypothalamic dysfunction.
- **Transcranial Magnetic Stimulation (TMS):** TMS uses magnetic fields to stimulate specific areas of the brain. It has been explored as a potential treatment for depression, anxiety, and memory impairments.
- **Cognitive-Behavioral Therapy (CBT):** CBT can help individuals develop coping strategies for stress, anxiety, and depression, which can indirectly impact hippocampal and hypothalamic function.

Stem Cell Therapies

- **Neural Stem Cell Transplantation:** The transplantation of neural stem cells into the brain has shown potential for repairing damaged tissue and promoting neurogenesis in animal models. Clinical trials are exploring the feasibility of this approach for treating neurodegenerative diseases like Alzheimer's and Parkinson's.
- **Induced Pluripotent Stem Cells (iPSCs):** iPSCs can be generated from adult cells and then differentiated into various cell types, including neurons. This technology offers a promising avenue for studying hippocampal and hypothalamic function and developing personalized therapies.

Lifestyle Interventions

- **Exercise:** Regular physical activity has been shown to have beneficial effects on brain health, including improving cognitive function and reducing stress.
- **Diet:** A healthy diet rich in nutrients can support brain health and reduce the risk of neurodegenerative diseases.
- **Stress Management:** Techniques such as mindfulness meditation, yoga, and deep breathing can help manage stress and reduce its negative impact on the hippocampus and hypothalamus.

Personalized Medicine

- **Genetic Testing:** Identifying genetic factors that contribute to hippocampal and hypothalamic dysfunction can help to tailor treatments to individual patients.
- **Precision Medicine:** By combining genetic information with clinical data and neuroimaging techniques, researchers can develop more personalized and effective therapeutic strategies.

Ethical Considerations

- **Consent and Safety:** Ensuring informed consent and minimizing risks associated with emerging therapeutic strategies is crucial.
- **Equity and Access:** Efforts should be made to ensure that new treatments are accessible to all patients, regardless of socioeconomic status or geographic location.

Conclusion

The field of hippocampal and hypothalamic research is rapidly evolving, and emerging therapeutic strategies hold great promise for improving the lives of individuals with brain disorders. By combining innovative technologies, personalized medicine, and lifestyle interventions, researchers can develop more effective and targeted treatments for conditions such as memory impairments, mood disorders, and neurodegenerative diseases.

Chapter 23: Emerging Therapeutic Strategies for Hippocampal and Hypothalamic Dysfunction

Introduction

The hippocampus and hypothalamus, two critical brain regions involved in memory, emotion, and homeostasis, are implicated in a variety of neurological and psychiatric disorders. As our understanding of these structures and their functions continues to evolve, so too do the therapeutic strategies being developed to address associated conditions. This chapter will explore some of the most promising emerging therapeutic approaches targeting hippocampal and hypothalamic dysfunction.

Pharmacological Interventions

- **Neuroprotective Agents:** Research is focused on identifying compounds that can protect hippocampal and hypothalamic neurons from damage. This includes exploring the potential of antioxidants, anti-inflammatory agents, and neurotrophic factors.
- **Modulation of Neurotransmitters:** Targeting neurotransmitters involved in hippocampal and hypothalamic function, such as glutamate, GABA, dopamine, and serotonin, holds promise for treating disorders like depression, anxiety, and memory impairments.
- **Hormone Therapies:** Manipulating hormonal pathways, particularly the hypothalamic-pituitary-adrenal (HPA) axis, is being investigated for conditions like stress-related disorders and metabolic disturbances.

Non-Pharmacological Interventions

- **Brain-Computer Interfaces (BCIs):** BCIs aim to restore lost functions or enhance cognitive abilities by establishing communication between the brain and external devices. They may be particularly useful for treating memory impairments or motor deficits associated with hippocampal and hypothalamic dysfunction.
- **Deep Brain Stimulation (DBS):** This technique involves implanting electrodes into specific brain regions to deliver electrical stimulation. DBS has shown promise in treating conditions like depression, obsessive-compulsive disorder, and Parkinson's disease, which often involve hippocampal and hypothalamic dysfunction.
- **Transcranial Magnetic Stimulation (TMS):** TMS uses magnetic fields to stimulate specific areas of the brain. It has been explored as a potential treatment for depression, anxiety, and memory impairments.
- **Cognitive-Behavioral Therapy (CBT):** CBT can help individuals develop coping strategies for stress, anxiety, and depression, which can indirectly impact hippocampal and hypothalamic function.

Stem Cell Therapies

- **Neural Stem Cell Transplantation:** The transplantation of neural stem cells into the brain has shown potential for repairing damaged tissue and promoting neurogenesis in animal models. Clinical trials are exploring the feasibility of this approach for treating neurodegenerative diseases like Alzheimer's and Parkinson's.
- **Induced Pluripotent Stem Cells (iPSCs):** iPSCs can be generated from adult cells and then differentiated into various cell types, including neurons. This technology offers a promising avenue for studying hippocampal and hypothalamic function and developing personalized therapies.

Lifestyle Interventions

- **Exercise:** Regular physical activity has been shown to have beneficial effects on brain health, including improving cognitive function and reducing stress.
- **Diet:** A healthy diet rich in nutrients can support brain health and reduce the risk of neurodegenerative diseases.
- **Stress Management:** Techniques such as mindfulness meditation, yoga, and deep breathing can help manage stress and reduce its negative impact on the hippocampus and hypothalamus.

Personalized Medicine

- **Genetic Testing:** Identifying genetic factors that contribute to hippocampal and hypothalamic dysfunction can help to tailor treatments to individual patients.
- **Precision Medicine:** By combining genetic information with clinical data and neuroimaging techniques, researchers can develop more personalized and effective therapeutic strategies.

Ethical Considerations

- **Consent and Safety:** Ensuring informed consent and minimizing risks associated with emerging therapeutic strategies is crucial.
- **Equity and Access:** Efforts should be made to ensure that new treatments are accessible to all patients, regardless of socioeconomic status or geographic location.

Conclusion

The field of hippocampal and hypothalamic research is rapidly evolving, and emerging therapeutic strategies hold great promise for improving the lives of individuals with brain disorders. By combining innovative technologies, personalized medicine, and lifestyle interventions, researchers can develop more effective and targeted treatments for conditions such as memory impairments, mood disorders, and neurodegenerative diseases.

Chapter 24: Future Directions and Emerging Research

Introduction

The hippocampus and hypothalamus, two key structures within the limbic system, continue to be the subject of intense research. Advances in neuroscience technology and methodologies have opened up new avenues for exploring the complex interactions between these regions and their roles in various cognitive and physiological functions. This chapter will delve into the exciting field of emerging research, highlighting potential future directions and the implications for understanding the brain and developing novel therapeutic strategies.

Neuroimaging Techniques

- **Advanced MRI Techniques:** Diffusion tensor imaging (DTI) and functional MRI (fMRI) have provided invaluable insights into the structural and functional connectivity of the hippocampus and hypothalamus. Future advancements in these techniques may allow for even more precise mapping and analysis of neural networks.
- **Optogenetics:** This revolutionary technique enables researchers to control the activity of specific neurons using light. Optogenetics can be used to study the causal relationships between hippocampal and hypothalamic activity and behavior.
- **In Vivo Electrophysiology:** Techniques such as single-unit recording and calcium imaging allow for the precise measurement of neuronal activity in real time, providing valuable information about the neural circuits underlying hippocampal and hypothalamic functions.

Molecular and Cellular Biology

- **Epigenetics:** Epigenetic modifications, such as DNA methylation and histone acetylation, can alter gene expression and influence brain function. Research is exploring the role of epigenetics in regulating hippocampal and hypothalamic development and plasticity.
- **Neurogenesis:** The hippocampus is known for its neurogenesis, the process of generating new neurons. Understanding the factors that regulate neurogenesis may provide insights into potential therapeutic strategies for brain disorders.
- **Neurotransmitters and Receptors:** Advances in understanding the role of neurotransmitters and receptors in hippocampal and hypothalamic function are ongoing. Identifying novel targets for therapeutic intervention may lead to the development of more effective treatments.

Computational Neuroscience

- **Neural Networks:** Computational models of the hippocampus and hypothalamus are being developed to simulate their complex interactions and predict their behavior. These models can help to test hypotheses and generate new insights.
- **Machine Learning:** Machine learning algorithms can be used to analyze large datasets of neural activity and identify patterns that may be relevant to hippocampal and hypothalamic function.

Therapeutic Implications

- **Personalized Medicine:** Advances in neuroscience may enable the development of personalized treatments based on an individual's unique genetic makeup and brain function.
- **Brain-Computer Interfaces:** Brain-computer interfaces (BCIs) may be used to restore lost functions or enhance cognitive abilities in individuals with brain disorders or injuries.
- **Neuroprosthetic Devices:** Neuroprosthetic devices can be implanted into the brain to stimulate specific regions and improve function. These devices may be used to treat conditions such as depression, anxiety, and memory disorders.

Ethical Considerations

- **Privacy and Consent:** As neuroscience research advances, it is essential to address ethical concerns related to data privacy and informed consent.
- **Dual-Use Concerns:** The potential for misuse of neuroscience technology, such as in developing mind-control weapons, raises ethical questions.

Conclusion

The field of neuroscience is rapidly evolving, and the hippocampus and hypothalamus remain at the forefront of research. Future advancements in technology and methodologies will undoubtedly lead to new discoveries and insights into the complex interactions between these brain regions and their roles in behavior and disease. By addressing ethical concerns and harnessing the potential of emerging technologies, researchers can continue to make significant contributions to our understanding of the brain and develop innovative therapeutic strategies.

Chapter 25: Future Directions and Emerging Research

Introduction

The hippocampus and hypothalamus, two key structures within the limbic system, continue to be the subject of intense research. Advances in neuroscience technology and methodologies have opened up new avenues for exploring the complex interactions between these regions and their roles in various cognitive and physiological functions. This chapter will delve into the exciting field of emerging research, highlighting potential future directions and the implications for understanding the brain and developing novel therapeutic strategies.

Neuroimaging Techniques

- **Advanced MRI Techniques:** Diffusion tensor imaging (DTI) and functional MRI (fMRI) have provided invaluable insights into the structural and functional connectivity of the hippocampus and hypothalamus. Future advancements in these techniques may allow for even more precise mapping and analysis of neural networks.
- **Optogenetics:** This revolutionary technique enables researchers to control the activity of specific neurons using light. Optogenetics can be used to study the causal relationships between hippocampal and hypothalamic activity and behavior.
- **In Vivo Electrophysiology:** Techniques such as single-unit recording and calcium imaging allow for the precise measurement of neuronal activity in real time, providing valuable information about the neural circuits underlying hippocampal and hypothalamic functions.

Molecular and Cellular Biology

- **Epigenetics:** Epigenetic modifications, such as DNA methylation and histone acetylation, can alter gene expression and influence brain function. Research is exploring the role of epigenetics in regulating hippocampal and hypothalamic development and plasticity.
- **Neurogenesis:** The hippocampus is known for its neurogenesis, the process of generating new neurons. Understanding the factors that regulate neurogenesis may provide insights into potential therapeutic strategies for brain disorders.
- **Neurotransmitters and Receptors:** Advances in understanding the role of neurotransmitters and receptors in hippocampal and hypothalamic function are ongoing. Identifying novel targets for therapeutic intervention may lead to the development of more effective treatments.

Computational Neuroscience

- **Neural Networks:** Computational models of the hippocampus and hypothalamus are being developed to simulate their complex interactions and predict their behavior. These models can help to test hypotheses and generate new insights.
- **Machine Learning:** Machine learning algorithms can be used to analyze large datasets of neural activity and identify patterns that may be relevant to hippocampal and hypothalamic function.

Therapeutic Implications

- **Personalized Medicine:** Advances in neuroscience may enable the development of personalized treatments based on an individual's unique genetic makeup and brain function.
- **Brain-Computer Interfaces:** Brain-computer interfaces (BCIs) may be used to restore lost functions or enhance cognitive abilities in individuals with brain disorders or injuries.
- **Neuroprosthetic Devices:** Neuroprosthetic devices can be implanted into the brain to stimulate specific regions and improve function. These devices may be used to treat conditions such as depression, anxiety, and memory disorders.

Ethical Considerations

- **Privacy and Consent:** As neuroscience research advances, it is essential to address ethical concerns related to data privacy and informed consent.
- **Dual-Use Concerns:** The potential for misuse of neuroscience technology, such as in developing mind-control weapons, raises ethical questions.

Conclusion

The field of neuroscience is rapidly evolving, and the hippocampus and hypothalamus remain at the forefront of research. Future advancements in technology and methodologies will undoubtedly lead to new discoveries and insights into the complex interactions between these brain regions and their roles in behavior and disease. By addressing ethical concerns and harnessing the potential of emerging technologies, researchers can continue to make significant contributions to our understanding of the brain and develop innovative therapeutic strategies.

Chapter 1: The Pineal Gland: A Brief Overview

Introduction

The pineal gland, a small, pea-sized structure nestled deep within the brain, has captivated the human imagination for centuries. Often referred to as the "third eye," it has been associated with spiritual enlightenment, intuition, and even psychic abilities. While these mystical connotations have persisted, modern scientific research has shed light on the pineal gland's essential role in regulating various biological functions. In this chapter, we will explore the anatomy, physiology, and historical significance of the pineal gland, laying the foundation for our journey to understand its profound impact on human consciousness.

Anatomy and Location

The pineal gland is situated in the center of the brain, near the thalamus and cerebellum. It is surrounded by cerebrospinal fluid, which provides protection and nourishment. Despite its small size, the pineal gland is a complex organ composed of pinealocytes, specialized cells that produce melatonin, a hormone crucial for regulating sleep-wake cycles.

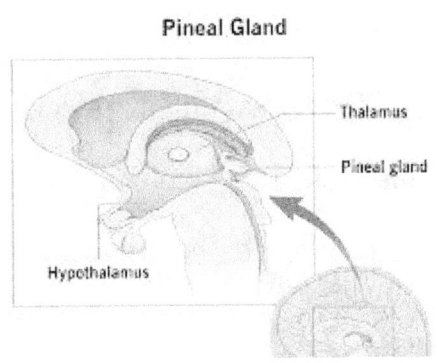

Opens in a new window my.clevelandclinic.org

pineal gland in the brain

Physiology and Function

The pineal gland's primary function is to produce melatonin in response to light and dark cues. During the day, when light levels are high, melatonin production is suppressed. As darkness falls, the pineal gland begins to secrete melatonin, signaling the body to prepare for sleep. Melatonin plays a vital role in regulating circadian rhythms, ensuring that we sleep at the right time and for the appropriate duration.

In addition to its role in sleep regulation, the pineal gland may also be involved in other biological processes. Some studies suggest that it may play a role in mood regulation, immune function, and even reproductive development. However, more research is needed to fully understand the pineal gland's complex functions.

Historical Significance

The pineal gland has been a subject of fascination and speculation for centuries. Ancient civilizations, such as the Egyptians, Greeks, and Hindus, believed that the pineal gland was a spiritual center, associated with intuition, enlightenment, and the connection to higher consciousness. The philosopher René Descartes famously referred to the pineal gland as the "seat of the soul."

In more recent times, the pineal gland has been linked to various New Age and spiritual movements. Some proponents of these movements believe that the pineal gland can be activated to unlock hidden potentials, such as psychic abilities and spiritual enlightenment. While these claims are largely unsubstantiated, they highlight the enduring fascination with the pineal gland and its potential significance beyond its biological functions.

Conclusion

The pineal gland is a small but essential organ that plays a crucial role in regulating sleep-wake cycles and other biological functions. Its historical significance and association with spiritual enlightenment have captivated the human imagination for centuries. As we delve deeper into the mysteries of the pineal gland, we may uncover even more profound insights into its role in human consciousness and well-being.

Chapter 2: The Pineal Gland and Light

Introduction

The pineal gland, a small, pea-sized structure located deep within the brain, has long been shrouded in mystery. While its primary function is to regulate sleep-wake cycles through the production of melatonin, recent research has revealed its intricate relationship with light. Light, a fundamental aspect of our environment, exerts a profound influence on the pineal gland, shaping our circadian rhythms and potentially impacting our overall health and well-being. In this chapter, we will explore the complex interplay between the pineal gland and light, examining how light exposure affects melatonin production, circadian rhythms, and other biological processes.

The Pineal Gland and Melatonin Production

The pineal gland's primary function is to produce melatonin, a hormone that regulates our sleep-wake cycles. Melatonin production is influenced by light exposure. During the day, when light levels are high, melatonin production is suppressed. This allows us to stay awake and alert. As darkness falls, the pineal gland begins to secrete melatonin, signaling the body to prepare for sleep. The amount of melatonin produced is directly related to the intensity and duration of darkness.

The retina, a light-sensitive tissue at the back of the eye, plays a crucial role in transmitting light information to the pineal gland. Specialized cells in the retina, called photoreceptors, detect light and send signals to the suprachiasmatic nucleus (SCN), a region of the brain that regulates circadian rhythms. The SCN, in turn, communicates with the pineal gland, influencing melatonin production.

The Impact of Light on Circadian Rhythms

Circadian rhythms are approximately 24-hour biological cycles that regulate various physiological processes, including sleep, wakefulness, body temperature, and hormone production. Light plays a vital role in synchronizing our circadian rhythms with the external environment. When we are exposed to bright light during the day, our circadian rhythms are aligned with the natural light-dark cycle. However, exposure to artificial light, particularly blue light emitted by electronic devices, can disrupt our circadian rhythms.

Blue light, which is similar to the light emitted by the sun, can suppress melatonin production, making it difficult to fall asleep. Excessive exposure to blue light at night can lead to sleep disturbances, fatigue, and other health problems. To maintain healthy circadian rhythms, it is important to minimize exposure to blue light in the evening and create a dark, relaxing environment for sleep.

The Role of Light in Other Biological Processes

In addition to regulating sleep-wake cycles, light may also influence other biological processes. Some studies suggest that light exposure can affect mood, cognitive function, and even the immune system. Exposure to sunlight can boost mood and reduce symptoms of depression. Light therapy, which involves exposure to bright light, has been used to treat seasonal affective disorder (SAD), a type of depression that occurs during the winter months.

Light may also play a role in regulating the immune system. Exposure to sunlight can increase the production of vitamin D, which is essential for immune function. Vitamin D deficiency has been linked to various health problems, including autoimmune diseases and infections.

Conclusion

The pineal gland and light are intricately linked, with light playing a critical role in regulating melatonin production, circadian rhythms, and other biological processes. Understanding the relationship between the pineal gland and light is essential for optimizing our health and well-being. By managing our exposure to light, we can improve our sleep quality, boost our mood, and support overall health.

Chapter 3: The Pineal Gland and Neurotransmitters

Introduction

The pineal gland, a small, pea-sized structure located deep within the brain, has long been associated with spiritual enlightenment and higher consciousness. While these mystical connotations have persisted, recent scientific research has revealed the pineal gland's essential role in regulating various biological functions. In addition to its role in producing melatonin, the pineal gland is also involved in the production and regulation of other neurotransmitters, chemical messengers that play a crucial role in brain function and behavior. In this chapter, we will explore the pineal gland's connection to neurotransmitters, examining how these substances influence our mood, cognition, and overall well-being.

The Pineal Gland and Serotonin

Serotonin is a neurotransmitter that plays a vital role in mood regulation, appetite, sleep, and memory. It is often referred to as the "happiness hormone" because of its association with positive emotions. The pineal gland is involved in the production of serotonin, although the exact mechanisms are not fully understood. Some studies suggest that the pineal gland may produce a precursor to serotonin, which is then converted into serotonin in other areas of the brain.

Low levels of serotonin have been linked to depression, anxiety, and other mood disorders. Some antidepressant medications work by increasing serotonin levels in the brain. By understanding the pineal gland's role in serotonin production, we may be able to develop new strategies for treating these conditions.

The Pineal Gland and Dopamine

Dopamine is another neurotransmitter that plays a crucial role in brain function. It is involved in reward, motivation, pleasure, and movement. Dopamine is also essential for learning and memory. The pineal gland may play a role in regulating dopamine levels, although the exact mechanisms are not fully understood.

Dysregulation of dopamine levels has been implicated in various neurological and psychiatric disorders, including Parkinson's disease, schizophrenia, and addiction. By understanding the pineal gland's role in dopamine production, we may be able to develop new treatments for these conditions.

The Pineal Gland and Other Neurotransmitters

The pineal gland may also be involved in the production or regulation of other neurotransmitters, such as norepinephrine and GABA. Norepinephrine is a neurotransmitter that plays a role in arousal, attention, and stress response. GABA (gamma-aminobutyric acid) is the primary inhibitory neurotransmitter in the brain, and it plays a crucial role in regulating anxiety and sleep.

Research on the pineal gland's role in neurotransmitter production is ongoing. As our understanding of the pineal gland's functions continues to grow, we may discover even more connections between this small but essential organ and our brain health and behavior.

Conclusion

The pineal gland is not only involved in regulating sleep-wake cycles through the production of melatonin but also plays a role in the production and regulation of other neurotransmitters. These neurotransmitters, including serotonin, dopamine, norepinephrine, and GABA, are essential for brain function and behavior. By understanding the pineal gland's role in neurotransmitter production, we may be able to develop new strategies for treating various neurological and psychiatric disorders. As research continues, we may uncover even more fascinating connections between the pineal gland and our overall well-being.

Chapter 4: The Third Eye: A Concept Across Cultures

Introduction

The concept of the third eye has captivated the human imagination for millennia, appearing in ancient texts, religious traditions, and spiritual practices across the globe. While modern science has provided a biological explanation for the pineal gland, the third eye remains a potent symbol of spiritual enlightenment, intuition, and connection to a higher consciousness. In this chapter, we will explore the historical and cultural significance of the third eye, examining its representation in various traditions and its potential connection to the pineal gland.

The Third Eye in Ancient Civilizations

The third eye is a prominent symbol in many ancient civilizations. In Hinduism, the third eye is known as the Ajna chakra, located between the eyebrows. It is believed to be the seat of intuition, wisdom, and spiritual perception. In Buddhism, the third eye is associated with the Buddha's enlightenment and is often depicted as a radiant light emanating from the forehead.

The Egyptians also incorporated the third eye into their mythology and symbolism. The Eye of Horus, a powerful symbol of healing and protection, is often depicted with a single eye or a third eye on the forehead. The Eye of Horus was believed to have the power to restore sight and health.

The Third Eye in Religious Traditions

The third eye has also been a significant concept in various religious traditions. In Christianity, the third eye is sometimes associated with the Holy Spirit or the inner eye of faith. In Islam, the third eye is known as the "inner eye" and is believed to be a source of spiritual vision and enlightenment.

The Third Eye and the Pineal Gland

While the concept of the third eye has its roots in ancient traditions, there is growing interest in its potential connection to the pineal gland. Some proponents of this theory argue that the pineal gland is the physical manifestation of the third eye, serving as a gateway to spiritual enlightenment and higher consciousness.

However, the connection between the pineal gland and the third eye remains speculative. While the pineal gland plays a crucial role in regulating sleep-wake cycles and other biological functions, there is no scientific evidence to support the claim that it is a spiritual center or a gateway to higher consciousness.

The Third Eye as a Symbol of Spiritual Enlightenment

Regardless of its connection to the pineal gland, the third eye remains a powerful symbol of spiritual enlightenment and intuition. It represents the ability to see beyond the physical world and tap into a deeper level of consciousness. The third eye is often associated with qualities such as wisdom, compassion, and inner peace.

Conclusion

The concept of the third eye has been a source of fascination and inspiration for centuries, appearing in ancient civilizations, religious traditions, and spiritual practices across the globe. While its connection to the pineal gland remains speculative, the third eye continues to be a potent symbol of spiritual enlightenment and intuition. As we explore the mysteries of the pineal gland and the human mind, the third eye may offer valuable insights into the nature of consciousness and our place in the universe.

Chapter 5: The Third Eye and Intuition

Introduction

The concept of the third eye has captivated the human imagination for millennia, often associated with spiritual enlightenment, intuition, and a connection to higher consciousness. While the pineal gland, a small, pea-sized structure located deep within the brain, has been linked to the third eye, the relationship between the two remains speculative. In this chapter, we will explore the concept of intuition and its potential connection to the pineal gland, examining how intuition can be developed and cultivated.

What is Intuition?

Intuition, often described as a "gut feeling" or a "sixth sense," is a form of non-conscious knowing that allows us to make decisions or judgments without relying solely on conscious thought or rational analysis. Intuition can be a powerful tool, guiding us toward the right path, helping us to avoid mistakes, and providing insights that are often beyond our conscious understanding.

The Role of the Pineal Gland in Intuition

While there is no definitive scientific evidence linking the pineal gland directly to intuition, some proponents of this theory argue that the pineal gland may play a role in facilitating intuitive processes. They suggest that the pineal gland may act as a bridge between the conscious and unconscious mind, allowing us to access information that is not available to our conscious awareness.

However, it is important to note that intuition is a complex phenomenon that involves multiple brain regions and neural pathways. While the pineal gland may play a role in facilitating intuitive processes, it is unlikely to be the sole determinant of our intuitive abilities.

Developing Intuition

Intuition is a skill that can be developed and cultivated through practice and mindfulness. Here are some strategies for developing intuition:

- **Trust your gut feelings:** Pay attention to your instincts and trust your intuition. Even if your conscious mind is unsure, your intuition may be guiding you in the right direction.
- **Practice mindfulness:** Mindfulness involves paying attention to the present moment without judgment. By cultivating mindfulness, you can become more attuned to your inner thoughts and feelings, which can help you to develop your intuition.
-
- **Meditate:** Meditation can help to quiet the mind and improve your ability to access your intuition. There are many different types of meditation techniques, so find one that works best for you.
- **Spend time in nature:** Spending time in nature can help to connect you with your intuition. The natural world can be a source of inspiration and guidance.
- **Keep a journal:** Journaling can help you to track your intuitive insights and patterns. Over time, you may begin to recognize recurring themes and patterns in your intuition.

The Benefits of Intuition

Developing your intuition can have many benefits, including:

- **Improved decision-making:** Intuition can help you to make better decisions, even when you don't have all the information.
- **Increased creativity:** Intuition can be a source of inspiration and creativity, helping you to come up with new ideas and solutions.
- **Enhanced emotional well-being:** Intuition can help you to connect with your emotions and develop a greater sense of emotional intelligence.
- **Spiritual growth:** Intuition can be a powerful tool for spiritual growth and self-discovery.

Conclusion

Intuition is a valuable skill that can be developed and cultivated through practice and mindfulness. While the exact relationship between the pineal gland and intuition remains speculative, it is clear that intuition plays a vital role in our lives. By developing our intuitive abilities, we can tap into a deeper level of consciousness and live more fulfilling and meaningful lives.

Chapter 6: The Third Eye and Spiritual Awakening

Introduction

The concept of the third eye has captivated the human imagination for centuries, often associated with spiritual enlightenment, intuition, and a connection to higher consciousness. While the pineal gland, a small, pea-sized structure located deep within the brain, has been linked to the third eye, the relationship between the two remains speculative. In this chapter, we will explore the connection between the third eye and spiritual awakening, examining how the activation of the third eye can lead to profound transformations in consciousness and perception.

Spiritual Awakening: A Definition

Spiritual awakening is a personal journey of self-discovery and enlightenment that involves a shift in consciousness from a limited, ego-centered perspective to a more expansive, interconnected worldview. It can involve a deepening of spiritual beliefs, a heightened sense of intuition, and a greater connection to the divine or universal consciousness.

The Role of the Third Eye in Spiritual Awakening

Proponents of the third eye concept argue that the activation of the third eye is essential for spiritual awakening. They believe that the third eye serves as a gateway to higher consciousness, allowing us to access spiritual knowledge and wisdom that is beyond our ordinary perception.

While there is no scientific evidence to support the claim that the pineal gland is a spiritual center or a gateway to higher consciousness, the concept of the third eye can provide a valuable framework for understanding the spiritual dimensions of human experience.

The Stages of Spiritual Awakening

Spiritual awakening is often described as a journey that involves several stages. These stages may include:

- **Awakening:** The initial stage of spiritual awakening involves a sense of dissatisfaction or unfulfillment with one's current life. This may lead to a search for meaning and purpose.
- **Purification:** As individuals embark on their spiritual journey, they may experience a process of purification, involving the release of negative emotions, beliefs, and behaviors.
- **Illumination:** The stage of illumination is characterized by a profound shift in consciousness, often accompanied by a sense of peace, joy, and interconnectedness.
- **Integration:** The final stage of spiritual awakening involves integrating the insights and experiences gained during the journey into one's daily life.

Activating the Third Eye

While there is no one-size-fits-all approach to activating the third eye, there are various practices that can help to cultivate spiritual awareness and facilitate the process of awakening. These practices may include:

- **Meditation:** Meditation is a powerful tool for quieting the mind and connecting with your inner self. Regular meditation can help to develop intuition, expand consciousness, and facilitate spiritual growth.
- **Visualization:** Visualization involves creating mental images of your desired outcomes or spiritual experiences. By visualizing the activation of your third eye, you can help to manifest your intentions.
- **Energy healing:** Energy healing techniques, such as Reiki or Qigong, can help to balance your energy centers and promote spiritual healing.
- **Nature connection:** Spending time in nature can help to connect you with your inner self and the universal consciousness.

Conclusion

The concept of the third eye offers a valuable framework for understanding the spiritual dimensions of human experience. While the relationship between the pineal gland and the third eye remains speculative, the activation of the third eye can be a powerful catalyst for spiritual awakening and personal transformation. By engaging in practices such as meditation, visualization, energy healing, and nature connection, individuals can cultivate spiritual awareness and embark on a journey of self-discovery and enlightenment.

Chapter 7: Detoxifying the Pineal Gland

Introduction

The pineal gland, a small, pea-sized structure located deep within the brain, has been a subject of fascination and speculation for centuries. While its primary function is to regulate sleep-wake cycles, it has also been associated with spiritual enlightenment and higher consciousness. In recent years, there has been growing interest in the idea that the pineal gland may become calcified over time, hindering its function and potentially contributing to various health problems. In this chapter, we will explore the concept of pineal gland calcification, its potential causes and consequences, and strategies for detoxifying the pineal gland.

Pineal Gland Calcification: A Growing Concern

The presence of calcium deposits in the pineal gland, known as calcification, is a common occurrence. As we age, the pineal gland gradually accumulates calcium oxalate crystals, which can reduce its size and interfere with its function. While the exact causes of pineal gland calcification are not fully understood, several factors may contribute to its development, including:

- **Aging:** Calcification is more common in older individuals, suggesting that it is a natural part of the aging process.
- **Fluoride exposure:** Some studies have suggested that exposure to fluoride, a common ingredient in drinking water and dental products, may contribute to pineal gland calcification.
- **Diet:** A diet high in processed foods and refined sugars may also contribute to calcification.
- **Environmental factors:** Exposure to toxins and pollutants may also play a role in pineal gland calcification.

The Consequences of Pineal Gland Calcification

The consequences of pineal gland calcification are not fully understood, but it is believed that it can interfere with the pineal gland's ability to produce melatonin, a hormone that regulates sleep-wake cycles. Reduced melatonin production can lead to sleep disturbances, mood disorders, and other health problems. Additionally, some proponents of the third eye concept argue that pineal gland calcification can hinder the development of intuition and spiritual awareness.

Strategies for Detoxifying the Pineal Gland

While there is no definitive scientific evidence to support the claim that the pineal gland can be detoxified, there are several strategies that may help to improve its function and reduce the risk of calcification. These strategies include:

- **Reducing fluoride exposure:** This can be achieved by filtering your drinking water, using fluoride-free toothpaste, and avoiding fluoridated products.
- **Eating a healthy diet:** A diet rich in fruits, vegetables, and whole grains can help to reduce inflammation and support overall health.
- **Limiting sugar intake:** Excessive sugar consumption has been linked to various health problems, including inflammation and oxidative stress.
- **Exercising regularly:** Regular physical activity can help to improve circulation and promote overall health.
- **Managing stress:** Chronic stress can contribute to inflammation and other health problems. Effective stress management techniques, such as meditation, yoga, or deep breathing exercises, can help to reduce stress and promote relaxation.

Conclusion

Pineal gland calcification is a common occurrence, but it may have negative consequences for sleep, mood, and overall health. While there is no definitive cure for pineal gland calcification, several strategies can help to reduce its risk and improve the pineal gland's function. By adopting a healthy lifestyle, reducing fluoride exposure, and managing stress, individuals can take steps to support the health of their pineal gland and promote optimal well-being.

Chapter 8: Nutrition for Pineal Gland Health

Introduction

The pineal gland, a small, pea-sized structure located deep within the brain, plays a crucial role in regulating sleep-wake cycles and other biological functions. While its exact role in spiritual enlightenment and higher consciousness remains a subject of debate, there is growing evidence that the pineal gland's health can be influenced by various factors, including nutrition. In this chapter, we will explore the relationship between nutrition and pineal gland health, examining the specific nutrients that can support its function and reduce the risk of calcification.

The Role of Antioxidants

Antioxidants are substances that protect cells from damage caused by harmful molecules known as free radicals. Free radicals can contribute to a variety of health problems, including inflammation, chronic diseases, and premature aging. Some research suggests that antioxidants may also play a role in protecting the pineal gland from damage and promoting its optimal function.

Foods rich in antioxidants include:

- **Fruits and vegetables:** Berries, dark leafy greens, and citrus fruits are particularly high in antioxidants.
- **Nuts and seeds:** Almonds, walnuts, and sunflower seeds are excellent sources of antioxidants.
- **Whole grains:** Whole grains, such as brown rice, quinoa, and oats, are rich in antioxidants and fiber.
- **Dark chocolate:** Dark chocolate with a high cocoa content is a good source of antioxidants.
- **Herbs and spices:** Turmeric, ginger, and cinnamon are known for their antioxidant properties.

The Importance of Omega-3 Fatty Acids

Omega-3 fatty acids are essential nutrients that the body cannot produce on its own. They must be obtained from food. Omega-3 fatty acids have been shown to have numerous health benefits, including reducing inflammation, improving heart health, and supporting brain function. Some research suggests that omega-3 fatty acids may also play a role in protecting the pineal gland from damage and promoting its optimal function.

Good sources of omega-3 fatty acids include:

- **Fatty fish:** Salmon, mackerel, sardines, and tuna are excellent sources of omega-3 fatty acids.
- **Flaxseed:** Flaxseed is a rich source of alpha-linolenic acid (ALA), a plant-based omega-3 fatty acid.
- **Chia seeds:** Chia seeds are also a good source of ALA.
- **Walnuts:** Walnuts are a rich source of omega-3 fatty acids.

The Role of Vitamin D

Vitamin D is essential for bone health, but it also plays a role in other biological functions, including immune function and mood regulation. Some research suggests that vitamin D deficiency may be linked to pineal gland calcification. Therefore, it is important to ensure that you are getting enough vitamin D.

The best source of vitamin D is sunlight exposure. However, if you have limited sun exposure, you can also obtain vitamin D from fortified foods, such as milk, yogurt, and orange juice.

The Importance of Hydration

Staying hydrated is essential for overall health, and it may also be important for pineal gland health. Dehydration can lead to a variety of health problems, including fatigue, headaches, and constipation. It may also contribute to inflammation and oxidative stress, which can damage the pineal gland.

Conclusion

Nutrition plays a crucial role in supporting pineal gland health. By consuming a diet rich in antioxidants, omega-3 fatty acids, vitamin D, and staying hydrated, individuals can help to protect the pineal gland from damage and promote its optimal function. While more research is needed to fully understand the relationship between nutrition and pineal gland health, the evidence suggests that a healthy diet can be a valuable tool for supporting overall well-being.

Chapter 9: Meditation and Mindfulness for Pineal Gland Activation

Introduction

The pineal gland, a small, pea-sized structure located deep within the brain, has long been associated with spiritual enlightenment and higher consciousness. While its exact role in these phenomena remains a subject of debate, there is growing interest in the idea that the pineal gland can be activated through various practices, including meditation and mindfulness. In this chapter, we will explore the connection between meditation and mindfulness and the pineal gland, examining how these practices can help to enhance spiritual awareness and promote the activation of the third eye.

The Benefits of Meditation and Mindfulness

Meditation and mindfulness are ancient practices that have been shown to have numerous benefits for physical and mental health. These benefits include:

- **Reduced stress and anxiety:** Meditation and mindfulness can help to reduce stress and anxiety by calming the mind and promoting relaxation.
- **Improved focus and concentration:** Regular meditation can enhance focus and concentration by improving attention span and reducing distractions.
- **Enhanced emotional well-being:** Meditation and mindfulness can help to regulate emotions and improve mood.
- **Improved sleep quality:** Meditation and mindfulness can help to improve sleep quality by reducing stress and promoting relaxation.
- **Boosted immune function:** Studies have shown that meditation and mindfulness can enhance immune function.

The Connection Between Meditation and Mindfulness and the Pineal Gland

While there is no direct scientific evidence linking meditation and mindfulness to the pineal gland, these practices may indirectly affect its function. Here are some possible mechanisms:

- **Reduced stress:** Chronic stress can contribute to inflammation and oxidative stress, which can damage the pineal gland. Meditation and mindfulness can help to reduce stress, thereby protecting the pineal gland from damage.
- **Improved sleep quality:** The pineal gland plays a crucial role in regulating sleep-wake cycles. By improving sleep quality, meditation and mindfulness can help to optimize the pineal gland's function.
- **Enhanced spiritual awareness:** Some proponents of the third eye concept argue that meditation and mindfulness can help to activate the third eye and enhance spiritual awareness.

Meditation Techniques for Pineal Gland Activation

There are many different types of meditation techniques, each with its own unique benefits. Here are a few examples:

- **Mindfulness meditation:** This involves paying attention to the present moment without judgment. It can be practiced by focusing on the breath, body sensations, or sounds.
- **Transcendental meditation:** This involves the use of a mantra or sound to quiet the mind and promote relaxation.
- **Guided meditation:** Guided meditations are led by a teacher or recording and can help to focus the mind and direct attention to specific areas of the body or mind.

Mindfulness Exercises for Pineal Gland Activation

In addition to meditation, mindfulness exercises can also be helpful for activating the pineal gland. These exercises involve paying attention to the present moment and cultivating a sense of awareness and presence. Here are a few examples of mindfulness exercises:

- **Body scan:** This involves focusing on different parts of the body and noticing any sensations or tensions.
- **Mindful eating:** This involves paying attention to the taste, texture, and smell of your food while eating.
- **Mindful walking:** This involves paying attention to your feet, the ground, and the sensations of walking.

Conclusion

Meditation and mindfulness are powerful tools for promoting spiritual growth and enhancing well-being. While there is no direct scientific evidence linking these practices to the pineal gland, they may indirectly affect its function by reducing stress, improving sleep quality, and enhancing spiritual awareness. By incorporating meditation and mindfulness into your daily routine, you can help to activate your third eye and unlock your full potential.

Chapter 10: Sound Therapy and Binaural Beats

Introduction

The pineal gland, a small, pea-sized structure located deep within the brain, has long been associated with spiritual enlightenment and higher consciousness. In recent years, there has been growing interest in the idea that the pineal gland can be activated through various practices, including sound therapy and binaural beats. In this chapter, we will explore the connection between sound and the pineal gland, examining how specific sound frequencies can influence brain activity and promote spiritual growth.

The Science of Sound Therapy

Sound therapy, also known as sound healing, is a therapeutic technique that involves the use of sound vibrations to promote relaxation, healing, and spiritual growth. Sound therapy can be used in various forms, including listening to music, chanting, or using specific sound frequencies.

The human body is composed of cells that vibrate at different frequencies. When exposed to specific sound frequencies, these cells can resonate and harmonize, promoting relaxation and healing. Sound therapy can also influence the brain's electrical activity, potentially affecting mood, cognition, and consciousness.

Binaural Beats: A Powerful Tool for Brainwave Entrainment

Binaural beats are auditory illusions created when two different tones are played simultaneously, one in each ear. The brain perceives the difference in frequency between the two tones as a third tone, known as the binaural beat. Binaural beats can be used to induce various states of consciousness, including relaxation, meditation, and creativity.

By listening to binaural beats, it is possible to entrain the brain's electrical activity to a specific frequency. This can have a profound impact on mood, cognition, and spiritual well-being. For example, listening to binaural beats in the theta frequency range (4-8 Hz) can promote relaxation and meditation, while listening to binaural beats in the alpha frequency range (8-12 Hz) can enhance creativity and problem-solving.

The Connection Between Sound Therapy and the Pineal Gland

While there is no direct scientific evidence linking sound therapy and binaural beats to the pineal gland, it is possible that these techniques may indirectly affect its function. Here are some potential mechanisms:

- **Reduced stress:** Sound therapy and binaural beats can help to reduce stress and anxiety, which can have a positive impact on overall health and well-being.
- **Improved sleep quality:** Sound therapy and binaural beats can help to improve sleep quality by promoting relaxation and reducing stress.
- **Enhanced spiritual awareness:** Some proponents of the third eye concept argue that sound therapy and binaural beats can help to activate the third eye and enhance spiritual awareness.

Using Sound Therapy and Binaural Beats to Activate the Pineal Gland

To use sound therapy and binaural beats to activate the pineal gland, it is important to choose the right frequencies and create a relaxing environment. Here are some tips:

- **Start with lower frequencies:** Begin with lower frequencies, such as theta or delta frequencies, to promote relaxation and meditation.
- **Gradually increase the frequency:** As you become more comfortable with sound therapy, you can gradually increase the frequency to explore different states of consciousness.
- **Create a peaceful environment:** Find a quiet, comfortable place to listen to sound therapy or binaural beats.
- **Use headphones:** Headphones can help to isolate the sound and enhance the experience.
- **Experiment with different frequencies:** There is no one-size-fits-all approach to sound therapy and binaural beats. Experiment with different frequencies to find what works best for you.

Conclusion

Sound therapy and binaural beats offer a powerful tool for promoting relaxation, healing, and spiritual growth. While there is no direct scientific evidence linking these techniques to the pineal gland, they may indirectly affect its function by reducing stress, improving sleep quality, and enhancing spiritual awareness. By incorporating sound therapy and binaural beats into your daily routine, you can help to activate your third eye and unlock your full potential.

Chapter 11: Crystal Therapy and Energy Healing

Introduction

The pineal gland, a small, pea-sized structure located deep within the brain, has long been associated with spiritual enlightenment and higher consciousness. In recent years, there has been growing interest in the idea that the pineal gland can be activated through various practices, including crystal therapy and energy healing. In this chapter, we will explore the connection between crystals and energy healing and the pineal gland, examining how these practices can help to enhance spiritual awareness and promote the activation of the third eye.

The Power of Crystals

Crystals are believed to possess unique energetic properties that can influence the human body and mind. Each crystal is thought to have its own specific vibrational frequency that can interact with our energy fields and promote healing and balance.

Some crystals that are believed to be particularly beneficial for the pineal gland include:

- **Amethyst:** Amethyst is often associated with spiritual awareness, intuition, and psychic abilities.
- **Third Eye:** This crystal is specifically named after the pineal gland and is believed to enhance its function.
- **Lapis Lazuli:** Lapis Lazuli is believed to stimulate the third eye and promote spiritual growth.
- **Fluorite:** Fluorite is believed to clear the mind, enhance concentration, and promote spiritual awareness.

Crystal Therapy Techniques

Crystal therapy involves the use of crystals to promote healing and balance. There are various techniques that can be used, including:

- **Crystal healing:** This involves placing crystals on the body or near the chakras to promote healing and balance.
- **Crystal meditation:** This involves holding or meditating with crystals to enhance spiritual awareness and intuition.
- **Crystal grids:** Crystal grids are arrangements of crystals that are believed to create a powerful energy field.

Energy Healing

Energy healing is a term used to describe a variety of practices that involve the manipulation of energy to promote healing and balance. Some popular energy healing techniques include:

- **Reiki:** Reiki is a Japanese technique for channeling universal life force energy.
- **Qigong:** Qigong is a Chinese practice that involves breathing exercises, meditation, and gentle movements.
- **Therapeutic touch:** Therapeutic touch involves the use of the hands to sense and manipulate energy fields.

The Connection Between Crystals, Energy Healing, and the Pineal Gland

While there is no scientific evidence to prove that crystals and energy healing can directly affect the pineal gland, these practices may indirectly influence its function. Here are some possible mechanisms:

- **Reduced stress:** Crystals and energy healing can help to reduce stress and anxiety, which can have a positive impact on overall health and well-being.
- **Enhanced spiritual awareness:** Many people believe that crystals and energy healing can help to enhance spiritual awareness and intuition.
- **Balanced energy fields:** By balancing the body's energy fields, crystals and energy healing may help to promote optimal health and function.

Using Crystals and Energy Healing to Activate the Pineal Gland

To use crystals and energy healing to activate the pineal gland, it is important to choose the right crystals and techniques. It is also important to have a clear intention and to approach these practices with an open mind.

Here are some tips for using crystals and energy healing to activate the pineal gland:

- **Choose the right crystals:** Research the properties of different crystals to find those that are most beneficial for the pineal gland.
- **Set a clear intention:** Before using crystals or energy healing, set a clear intention for what you want to achieve.
- **Relax and let go:** Allow yourself to relax and let go of any tension or stress during your crystal therapy or energy healing session.
- **Trust your intuition:** Trust your intuition to guide you in choosing the right crystals and techniques.

Conclusion

Crystals and energy healing offer a powerful tool for promoting spiritual growth and enhancing well-being. While there is no scientific evidence to prove that these practices can directly affect the pineal gland, they may indirectly influence its function by reducing stress, enhancing spiritual awareness, and balancing the body's energy fields. By incorporating crystals and energy healing into your daily routine, you can help to activate your third eye and unlock your full potential.

Chapter 12: Dream Interpretation and Lucid Dreaming

Introduction

The pineal gland, a small, pea-sized structure located deep within the brain, plays a crucial role in regulating sleep-wake cycles. It has also been associated with spiritual enlightenment and higher consciousness. In this chapter, we will explore the connection between the pineal gland, dreams, and lucid dreaming. We will examine the role of the pineal gland in dream formation and the potential benefits of lucid dreaming for personal growth and spiritual development.

The Pineal Gland and Dreams

The pineal gland is responsible for producing melatonin, a hormone that regulates sleep-wake cycles. Melatonin levels fluctuate throughout the night, influencing the stages of sleep. During REM sleep, the stage of sleep associated with vivid dreams, the pineal gland may play a role in shaping dream content.

Some researchers believe that the pineal gland may act as a gateway between the conscious and unconscious mind, allowing us to access information and experiences that are not available to our waking consciousness. This suggests that dreams may be a way for the pineal gland to process information and communicate with the conscious mind.

The Benefits of Lucid Dreaming

Lucid dreaming is a state of consciousness in which a person is aware that they are dreaming and can exert some degree of control over the dream's content. Lucid dreaming can be a powerful tool for personal growth and spiritual development. Some of the potential benefits of lucid dreaming include:

- **Improved creativity:** Lucid dreaming can enhance creativity by allowing individuals to explore new ideas and possibilities in a dreamlike state.
- **Enhanced problem-solving:** Lucid dreaming can help to solve problems and find creative solutions by allowing individuals to explore different perspectives and scenarios.
- **Personal growth:** Lucid dreaming can facilitate personal growth by providing opportunities for self-discovery and spiritual exploration.
- **Healing and transformation:** Lucid dreaming can be used as a tool for healing and transformation by addressing emotional issues and limiting beliefs.

Techniques for Achieving Lucid Dreaming

There are several techniques that can be used to increase the likelihood of achieving lucid dreaming. These techniques include:

- **Reality testing:** Regularly throughout the day, ask yourself if you are dreaming. This can help to train your mind to recognize dream reality.
- **Mnemonic techniques:** Use mnemonics or affirmations to remind yourself to become lucid while dreaming.
- **Dream journaling:** Keeping a dream journal can help you to recall your dreams and identify patterns that may lead to lucid dreaming.
- **Wake-back-to-bed technique:** This involves waking up after a few hours of sleep, staying awake for a short period, and then returning to sleep. This can increase the likelihood of entering REM sleep and achieving lucid dreaming.

Conclusion

The pineal gland plays a crucial role in sleep and dreaming. Lucid dreaming can be a powerful tool for personal growth and spiritual development. By understanding the relationship between the pineal gland, dreams, and lucid dreaming, individuals can learn to harness the power of their dreams and unlock their full potential.

Chapter 13: Emerging Research and Scientific Discoveries

Introduction

The pineal gland, a small, pea-sized structure located deep within the brain, has long been a subject of fascination and speculation. While its primary function is to regulate sleep-wake cycles, it has also been associated with spiritual enlightenment and higher consciousness. In recent years, there has been a surge of scientific interest in the pineal gland, with new research shedding light on its role in various biological processes and its potential connection to human consciousness.

The Pineal Gland and Aging

As we age, the pineal gland undergoes changes that can affect its function. Studies have shown that the pineal gland calcifies over time, accumulating calcium deposits that can interfere with its ability to produce melatonin. This decline in melatonin production is associated with sleep disturbances, mood disorders, and other health problems.

However, recent research suggests that it may be possible to slow down the process of pineal gland calcification through lifestyle modifications, such as regular exercise, a healthy diet, and stress management. Additionally, some researchers are exploring the potential of using supplements and medications to improve pineal gland function in older adults.

The Pineal Gland and Neurodegenerative Diseases

The pineal gland may also play a role in neurodegenerative diseases, such as Alzheimer's disease and Parkinson's disease. Some studies have found that pineal gland dysfunction is associated with these conditions. While the exact mechanisms are not fully understood, it is possible that the pineal gland's role in regulating circadian rhythms and hormone production may be involved.

Researchers are investigating the potential of targeting the pineal gland to develop new treatments for neurodegenerative diseases. For example, some studies have explored the use of melatonin supplements to improve cognitive function in individuals with Alzheimer's disease.

The Pineal Gland and Meditation

Meditation has long been associated with spiritual enlightenment and higher consciousness. Recent research suggests that meditation may also have a positive impact on the pineal gland. Studies have shown that regular meditation can reduce stress, improve sleep quality, and enhance cognitive function. These benefits may be related to the pineal gland's role in regulating circadian rhythms and hormone production.

The Pineal Gland and Consciousness

The pineal gland's role in human consciousness remains a subject of speculation and debate. Some researchers believe that the pineal gland may act as a gateway to higher consciousness, connecting us to a universal source of energy and information. While there is no definitive scientific evidence to support this claim, the pineal gland's unique location and function suggest that it may play a role in shaping our subjective experience of reality.

Emerging Technologies and the Pineal Gland

As technology continues to advance, researchers are exploring new ways to study and manipulate the pineal gland. For example, brain imaging techniques, such as magnetic resonance imaging (MRI) and positron emission tomography (PET), are being used to investigate the structure and function of the pineal gland. Additionally, researchers are developing new drugs and therapies that may target the pineal gland to treat various health conditions.

Conclusion

The pineal gland is a complex organ with a multifaceted role in human health and consciousness. As research continues to advance, we are gaining a deeper understanding of its functions and its potential connection to various biological processes. While the pineal gland's role in spiritual enlightenment and higher consciousness remains a subject of debate, it is clear that this small but essential organ plays a vital role in our lives.

Chapter 14: The Ethical Implications of Pineal Gland Activation

Introduction

The pineal gland, a small, pea-sized structure located deep within the brain, has long been associated with spiritual enlightenment and higher consciousness. In recent years, there has been growing interest in the idea that the pineal gland can be activated through various practices, including meditation, energy healing, and the use of specific substances. However, as our understanding of the pineal gland's role in human consciousness and behavior continues to evolve, it is important to consider the ethical implications of pineal gland activation.

The Potential Benefits and Risks of Pineal Gland Activation

Proponents of pineal gland activation argue that it can lead to a variety of benefits, including:

- Enhanced spiritual awareness and intuition
- Increased creativity and problem-solving abilities
- Improved mental and emotional health
- A deeper connection to the universe and a sense of meaning and purpose

However, there are also potential risks associated with pineal gland activation. These risks may include:

- **Unintended side effects:** Some practices or substances that are used to activate the pineal gland may have unintended side effects, such as hallucinations, anxiety, or changes in mood.
- **Ethical dilemmas:** The pursuit of spiritual enlightenment and higher consciousness can raise ethical questions, particularly when it involves the use of substances or practices that may be harmful or addictive.
- **Social implications:** The activation of the pineal gland may lead to changes in social behavior and relationships, which could have both positive and negative consequences.

The Role of Science and Ethics in Pineal Gland Research

As research into the pineal gland continues to advance, it is essential to approach the topic with a balanced perspective that takes into account both the potential benefits and risks. Scientists and researchers have a responsibility to conduct ethical research that safeguards the well-being of participants and avoids exploitation.

It is also important to consider the ethical implications of promoting pineal gland activation. While it is important to encourage personal growth and spiritual development, it is also crucial to ensure that individuals are informed about the potential risks and benefits of these practices.

Ethical Considerations for Individuals Pursuing Pineal Gland Activation

Individuals who are interested in pursuing pineal gland activation should be aware of the potential risks and benefits. They should also consider the following ethical considerations:

- **Informed consent:** Individuals should be fully informed about the potential risks and benefits of any practices or substances they intend to use to activate the pineal gland.
- **Personal responsibility:** Individuals should take responsibility for their own well-being and avoid engaging in practices that may be harmful or addictive.
- **Respect for others:** Individuals should be mindful of the potential impact of their spiritual practices on others and avoid imposing their beliefs on others.

Conclusion

The pineal gland is a fascinating organ with the potential to unlock new levels of consciousness and human potential. However, it is essential to approach the topic of pineal gland activation with caution and consider the ethical implications involved. By understanding the potential benefits and risks, and by engaging in ethical practices, individuals can safely explore the mysteries of the pineal gland and embark on a journey of spiritual growth and self-discovery.

Chapter 15: Conclusion: Embracing the Power of the Pineal Gland

Introduction

In this comprehensive exploration of the pineal gland, we have delved into its anatomical structure, physiological functions, and historical significance. We have examined its role in regulating sleep-wake cycles, producing neurotransmitters, and potentially influencing human consciousness. We have also explored the concept of the third eye and its connection to the pineal gland, as well as various practices and techniques for activating and balancing this enigmatic organ.

Key Takeaways

Throughout this book, we have covered a wide range of topics related to the pineal gland, including:

- The pineal gland's role in melatonin production and sleep-wake cycles
- The impact of light on pineal gland function
- The pineal gland's involvement in neurotransmitter production
- The historical and cultural significance of the third eye
- Techniques for activating the pineal gland, such as meditation, energy healing, and sound therapy
- The ethical implications of pineal gland activation

Embracing the Power of the Pineal Gland

The pineal gland is a complex and fascinating organ with the potential to profoundly influence our lives. By understanding its role in human health and consciousness, we can take steps to optimize its function and unlock our full potential.

Here are some key takeaways for embracing the power of the pineal gland:

- **Prioritize sleep:** Ensure you get adequate sleep in a dark, quiet environment to support healthy melatonin production.
- **Manage light exposure:** Minimize exposure to blue light from electronic devices before bed and spend time in natural light during the day.
- **Nourish your body:** Consume a healthy diet rich in antioxidants, omega-3 fatty acids, and vitamin D to support pineal gland health.
- **Reduce stress:** Chronic stress can negatively impact the pineal gland. Practice stress management techniques such as meditation, yoga, or deep breathing.
- **Explore spiritual practices:** Engage in meditation, mindfulness, energy healing, or other spiritual practices to connect with your inner self and activate your third eye.
- **Be mindful of ethical considerations:** Approach pineal gland activation with caution and consider the potential risks and benefits.

A Call to Action

The journey to master the pineal gland is a personal one. It requires dedication, self-awareness, and a willingness to explore new possibilities. By incorporating the practices and techniques discussed in this book into your daily life, you can unlock the extraordinary potential of your pineal gland and embark on a transformative journey of self-discovery and spiritual growth.

Conclusion

The pineal gland is more than just a small, pea-sized structure in the brain. It is a gateway to deeper consciousness, a symbol of spiritual enlightenment, and a powerful tool for personal growth and transformation. By understanding and harnessing the power of the pineal gland, we can unlock our full potential and live more fulfilling and meaningful lives.

Chapter 16: The Pineal Gland and Aging

Introduction

The pineal gland, a small, pea-sized structure located deep within the brain, plays a crucial role in regulating sleep-wake cycles and other biological functions. As we age, the pineal gland undergoes changes that can affect its function. In this chapter, we will explore the relationship between the pineal gland and aging, examining how aging can affect pineal gland function and the potential consequences for health and well-being.

Age-Related Changes in the Pineal Gland

As we age, the pineal gland undergoes several changes, including:

- **Calcification:** The pineal gland gradually accumulates calcium deposits over time, which can reduce its size and interfere with its function.
- **Reduced melatonin production:** The pineal gland's ability to produce melatonin declines with age, leading to sleep disturbances and other health problems.
- **Changes in circadian rhythms:** Aging can disrupt circadian rhythms, making it more difficult to fall asleep and stay asleep.

The Consequences of Pineal Gland Aging

The decline in pineal gland function associated with aging can have several negative consequences, including:

- **Sleep disorders:** Insomnia, sleep apnea, and other sleep disorders are more common in older adults.
- **Mood disorders:** Depression and anxiety are more prevalent in older adults, and they may be linked to changes in pineal gland function.
- **Cognitive decline:** Some studies have suggested that pineal gland dysfunction may contribute to cognitive decline and dementia.
- **Increased risk of chronic diseases:** Pineal gland dysfunction may also be linked to an increased risk of chronic diseases, such as heart disease, stroke, and diabetes.

Strategies for Supporting Pineal Gland Health in Aging

While aging is a natural process that cannot be reversed, there are several strategies that can help to support pineal gland health and mitigate the negative consequences of aging:

- **Maintain a healthy lifestyle:** A healthy diet, regular exercise, and adequate sleep can help to support overall health and well-being, including pineal gland function.
- **Manage stress:** Chronic stress can contribute to pineal gland dysfunction. Effective stress management techniques, such as meditation, yoga, or deep breathing exercises, can help to reduce stress and promote relaxation.
- **Consider supplements:** Some supplements, such as melatonin and vitamin D, may be beneficial for supporting pineal gland function in older adults. However, it is important to consult with a healthcare provider before taking any supplements.
- **Seek medical attention:** If you are experiencing sleep disturbances, mood changes, or other symptoms that may be related to pineal gland dysfunction, it is important to see a healthcare provider for evaluation and treatment.

Conclusion

The pineal gland plays a crucial role in human health and well-being, and its function can decline with age. By understanding the relationship between the pineal gland and aging, and by taking steps to support pineal gland health, individuals can help to mitigate the negative consequences of aging and enjoy a healthier, more fulfilling life.

Chapter 17: The Pineal Gland and Extraterrestrial Intelligence

Introduction

The pineal gland, a small, pea-sized structure located deep within the brain, has long been associated with spiritual enlightenment and higher consciousness. In recent years, there has been a growing interest in the potential connection between the pineal gland and extraterrestrial intelligence (ETI). Some proponents of this theory argue that the pineal gland may serve as a gateway to communication with extraterrestrial beings or that it may be a biological device implanted by extraterrestrial civilizations. In this chapter, we will explore the relationship between the pineal gland and extraterrestrial intelligence, examining the evidence and arguments for and against this theory.

The Pineal Gland and UFO Sightings

One of the most common connections between the pineal gland and extraterrestrial intelligence is the association with UFO sightings. Some people believe that the pineal gland may be involved in facilitating contact with extraterrestrial beings or that it may be a target for extraterrestrial abduction. However, there is no scientific evidence to support these claims.

The Pineal Gland and Ancient Civilizations

The pineal gland has been a subject of fascination and speculation for centuries. Ancient civilizations, such as the Egyptians and Hindus, believed that the pineal gland was a spiritual center, associated with intuition, enlightenment, and the connection to higher consciousness. Some proponents of the extraterrestrial intelligence theory argue that ancient civilizations may have had knowledge of extraterrestrial beings and that the pineal gland played a role in facilitating communication with them.

The Pineal Gland and Neurotransmitters

The pineal gland plays a crucial role in the production of melatonin, a hormone that regulates sleep-wake cycles. Melatonin is also involved in the production of other neurotransmitters, such as serotonin and dopamine, which are essential for brain function and behavior. Some proponents of the extraterrestrial intelligence theory argue that the pineal gland may be capable of producing neurotransmitters that allow us to communicate with extraterrestrial beings.

The Pineal Gland and Consciousness

The pineal gland's role in human consciousness remains a subject of debate. Some researchers believe that the pineal gland may act as a gateway to higher consciousness, connecting us to a universal source of energy and information. This has led some to speculate that the pineal gland may be involved in communication with extraterrestrial beings.

The Evidence for and Against the Extraterrestrial Intelligence Theory

There is no scientific evidence to support the claim that the pineal gland is involved in communication with extraterrestrial beings. While there have been numerous reports of UFO sightings and alleged encounters with extraterrestrial beings, these claims remain largely unsubstantiated.

Furthermore, the idea that the pineal gland is a biological device implanted by extraterrestrial civilizations is highly speculative and lacks any scientific basis.

Conclusion

The relationship between the pineal gland and extraterrestrial intelligence is a complex and controversial topic. While there is no scientific evidence to support the claim that the pineal gland is involved in communication with extraterrestrial beings, the pineal gland's role in human consciousness and behavior remains a fascinating area of research. As our understanding of the pineal gland continues to evolve, we may gain new insights into its potential connection to the mysteries of the universe.

Chapter 18: The Pineal Gland and the Collective Consciousness

Introduction

The pineal gland, a small, pea-sized structure located deep within the brain, has long been associated with spiritual enlightenment and higher consciousness. In recent years, there has been growing interest in the idea that the pineal gland may play a role in connecting us to a collective consciousness, a universal energy field that unites all living beings. In this chapter, we will explore the concept of collective consciousness and its potential relationship to the pineal gland.

Collective Consciousness: A Definition

Collective consciousness, also known as the global consciousness or the noosphere, is a hypothetical field of energy that connects all living beings. Proponents of this theory argue that we are all interconnected at a deeper level, sharing thoughts, emotions, and experiences.

The concept of collective consciousness has been explored by various philosophers, scientists, and spiritual leaders. Carl Jung, for example, believed that the collective consciousness was a shared pool of archetypal images and symbols that influence our thoughts and behaviors.

The Pineal Gland and Collective Consciousness

Some researchers believe that the pineal gland may play a role in connecting us to the collective consciousness. They argue that the pineal gland may be able to receive and transmit information from this universal energy field.

One potential mechanism for this connection is through the pineal gland's role in producing melatonin. Melatonin is a hormone that regulates sleep-wake cycles and has also been shown to have antioxidant properties. Some researchers believe that melatonin may also play a role in facilitating communication with the collective consciousness.

The Evidence for and Against the Collective Consciousness Theory

There is no definitive scientific evidence to support the existence of a collective consciousness. However, there are some anecdotal reports and personal experiences that suggest a connection between individuals and a universal energy field.

Some proponents of the collective consciousness theory argue that the synchronicity of events, such as coincidences and shared experiences, is evidence of a deeper connection between all living beings. Others point to the phenomenon of group consciousness, where large groups of people seem to be connected by a shared energy field.

Critics of the collective consciousness theory argue that these phenomena can be explained by other factors, such as chance, coincidence, or shared cultural beliefs. They also point out that there is no scientific evidence to support the existence of a universal energy field.

The Implications of Collective Consciousness

If the collective consciousness exists, it could have profound implications for our understanding of human consciousness and our place in the universe. It could suggest that we are all interconnected at a deeper level, sharing thoughts, emotions, and experiences. This could have implications for social, political, and environmental issues, as it suggests that our actions can have a ripple effect on the entire planet.

Conclusion

The concept of collective consciousness is a fascinating and controversial one. While there is no definitive scientific evidence to support its existence, it is a topic that continues to intrigue researchers and spiritual seekers alike. The pineal gland, with its unique role in human consciousness and its potential connection to higher states of awareness, may offer insights into the nature of collective consciousness. As our understanding of the pineal gland and the human mind continues to evolve, we may gain a deeper appreciation for the interconnectedness of all things.

Chapter 19: The Pineal Gland and the Collective Consciousness

Introduction

The pineal gland, a small, pea-sized structure located deep within the brain, has long been associated with spiritual enlightenment and higher consciousness. In recent years, there has been growing interest in the idea that the pineal gland may play a role in connecting us to a collective consciousness, a universal energy field that unites all living beings. In this chapter, we will explore the concept of collective consciousness and its potential relationship to the pineal gland.

Collective Consciousness: A Definition

Collective consciousness, also known as the global consciousness or the noosphere, is a hypothetical field of energy that connects all living beings. Proponents of this theory argue that we are all interconnected at a deeper level, sharing thoughts, emotions, and experiences.

The concept of collective consciousness has been explored by various philosophers, scientists, and spiritual leaders. Carl Jung, for example, believed that the collective consciousness was a shared pool of archetypal images and symbols that influence our thoughts and behaviors.

The Pineal Gland and Collective Consciousness

Some researchers believe that the pineal gland may play a role in connecting us to the collective consciousness. They argue that the pineal gland may be able to receive and transmit information from this universal energy field.

One potential mechanism for this connection is through the pineal gland's role in producing melatonin. Melatonin is a hormone that regulates sleep-wake cycles and has also been shown to have antioxidant properties. Some researchers believe that melatonin may also play a role in facilitating communication with the collective consciousness.

The Evidence for and Against the Collective Consciousness Theory

There is no definitive scientific evidence to support the existence of a collective consciousness. However, there are some anecdotal reports and personal experiences that suggest a connection between individuals and a universal energy field.

Some proponents of the collective consciousness theory argue that the synchronicity of events, such as coincidences and shared experiences, is evidence of a deeper connection between all living beings. Others point to the phenomenon of group consciousness, where large groups of people seem to be connected by a shared energy field.

Critics of the collective consciousness theory argue that these phenomena can be explained by other factors, such as chance, coincidence, or shared cultural beliefs. They also point out that there is no scientific evidence to support the existence of a universal energy field.

The Implications of Collective Consciousness

If the collective consciousness exists, it could have profound implications for our understanding of human consciousness and our place in the universe. It could suggest that we are all interconnected at a deeper level, sharing thoughts, emotions, and experiences. This could have implications for social, political, and environmental issues, as it suggests that our actions can have a ripple effect on the entire planet.

Conclusion

The concept of collective consciousness is a fascinating and controversial one. While there is no definitive scientific evidence to support its existence, it is a topic that continues to intrigue researchers and spiritual seekers alike. The pineal gland, with its unique role in human consciousness and its potential connection to higher states of awareness, may offer insights into the nature of collective consciousness. As our understanding of the pineal gland and the human mind continues to evolve, we may gain a deeper appreciation for the interconnectedness of all things.

Chapter 20: The Pineal Gland and Extraterrestrial Intelligence

Introduction

The pineal gland, a small, pea-sized structure located deep within the brain, has long been associated with spiritual enlightenment and higher consciousness. In recent years, there has been a growing interest in the idea that the pineal gland may play a role in connecting us to extraterrestrial intelligence (ETI). Some proponents of this theory argue that the pineal gland may serve as a gateway to communication with extraterrestrial beings or that it may be a biological device implanted by extraterrestrial civilizations. In this chapter, we will explore the relationship between the pineal gland and extraterrestrial intelligence, examining the evidence and arguments for and against this theory.

The Pineal Gland and UFO Sightings

One of the most common connections between the pineal gland and extraterrestrial intelligence is the association with UFO sightings. Some people believe that the pineal gland may be involved in facilitating contact with extraterrestrial beings or that it may be a target for extraterrestrial abduction. However, there is no scientific evidence to support these claims.

The Pineal Gland and Ancient Civilizations

The pineal gland has been a subject of fascination and speculation for centuries. Ancient civilizations, such as the Egyptians and Hindus, believed that the pineal gland was a spiritual center, associated with intuition, enlightenment, and the connection to higher consciousness. Some proponents of the extraterrestrial intelligence theory argue that ancient civilizations may have had knowledge of extraterrestrial beings and that the pineal gland played a role in facilitating communication with them.

The Pineal Gland and Neurotransmitters

The pineal gland plays a crucial role in the production of melatonin, a hormone that regulates sleep-wake cycles. Melatonin is also involved in the production of other neurotransmitters, such as serotonin and dopamine, which are essential for brain function and behavior. Some proponents of the extraterrestrial intelligence theory argue that the pineal gland may be capable of producing neurotransmitters that allow us to communicate with extraterrestrial beings.

The Pineal Gland and Consciousness

The pineal gland's role in human consciousness remains a subject of debate. Some researchers believe that the pineal gland may act as a gateway to higher consciousness, connecting us to a universal source of energy and information. This has led some to speculate that the pineal gland may be involved in communication with extraterrestrial beings.

The Evidence for and Against the Extraterrestrial Intelligence Theory

There is no scientific evidence to support the claim that the pineal gland is involved in communication with extraterrestrial beings. While there have been numerous reports of UFO sightings and alleged encounters with extraterrestrial beings, these claims remain largely unsubstantiated.

Furthermore, the idea that the pineal gland is a biological device implanted by extraterrestrial civilizations is highly speculative and lacks any scientific basis.

Conclusion

The relationship between the pineal gland and extraterrestrial intelligence is a complex and controversial topic. While there is no scientific evidence to support the claim that the pineal gland is involved in communication with extraterrestrial beings, the pineal gland's role in human consciousness and behavior remains a fascinating area of research. As our understanding of the pineal gland continues to evolve, we may gain new insights into its potential connection to the mysteries of the universe.

Chapter 21: The Pineal Gland and the Collective Consciousness

Introduction

The pineal gland, a small, pea-sized structure located deep within the brain, has long been associated with spiritual enlightenment and higher consciousness. In recent years, there has been growing interest in the idea that the pineal gland may play a role in connecting us to a collective consciousness, a universal energy field that unites all living beings. In this chapter, we will explore the concept of collective consciousness and its potential relationship to the pineal gland.

Collective Consciousness: A Definition

Collective consciousness, also known as the global consciousness or the noosphere, is a hypothetical field of energy that connects all living beings. Proponents of this theory argue that we are all interconnected at a deeper level, sharing thoughts, emotions, and experiences.

The concept of collective consciousness has been explored by various philosophers, scientists, and spiritual leaders. Carl Jung, for example, believed that the collective consciousness was a shared pool of archetypal images and symbols that influence our thoughts and behaviors.

The Pineal Gland and Collective Consciousness

Some researchers believe that the pineal gland may play a role in connecting us to the collective consciousness. They argue that the pineal gland may be able to receive and transmit information from this universal energy field.

One potential mechanism for this connection is through the pineal gland's role in producing melatonin. Melatonin is a hormone that regulates sleep-wake cycles and has also been shown to have antioxidant properties. Some researchers believe that melatonin may also play a role in facilitating communication with the collective consciousness.

The Evidence for and Against the Collective Consciousness Theory

There is no definitive scientific evidence to support the existence of a collective consciousness. However, there are some anecdotal reports and personal experiences that suggest a connection between individuals and a universal energy field.

Some proponents of the collective consciousness theory argue that the synchronicity of events, such as coincidences and shared experiences, is evidence of a deeper connection between all living beings. Others point to the phenomenon of group consciousness, where large groups of people seem to be connected by a shared energy field.

Critics of the collective consciousness theory argue that these phenomena can be explained by other factors, such as chance, coincidence, or shared cultural beliefs. They also point out that there is no scientific evidence to support the existence of a universal energy field.

The Implications of Collective Consciousness

If the collective consciousness exists, it could have profound implications for our understanding of human consciousness and our place in the universe. It could suggest that we are all interconnected at a deeper level, sharing thoughts, emotions, and experiences. This could have implications for social, political, and environmental issues, as it suggests that our actions can have a ripple effect on the entire planet.

Conclusion

The concept of collective consciousness is a fascinating and controversial one. While there is no definitive scientific evidence to support its existence, it is a topic that continues to intrigue researchers and spiritual seekers alike. The pineal gland, with its unique role in human consciousness and its potential connection to higher states of awareness, may offer insights into the nature of collective consciousness. As our understanding of the pineal gland and the human mind continues to evolve, we may gain a deeper appreciation for the interconnectedness of all things.

Chapter 22: The Pineal Gland and the Collective Consciousness

Introduction

The pineal gland, a small, pea-sized structure located deep within the brain, has long been associated with spiritual enlightenment and higher consciousness. In recent years, there has been growing interest in the idea that the pineal gland may play a role in connecting us to a collective consciousness, a universal energy field that unites all living beings. In this chapter, we will explore the concept of collective consciousness and its potential relationship to the pineal gland.

Collective Consciousness: A Definition

Collective consciousness, also known as the global consciousness or the noosphere, is a hypothetical field of energy that connects all living beings. Proponents of this theory argue that we are all interconnected at a deeper level, sharing thoughts, emotions, and experiences.

The concept of collective consciousness has been explored by various philosophers, scientists, and spiritual leaders. Carl Jung, for example, believed that the collective consciousness was a shared pool of archetypal images and symbols that influence our thoughts and behaviors.

The Pineal Gland and Collective Consciousness

Some researchers believe that the pineal gland may play a role in connecting us to the collective consciousness. They argue that the pineal gland may be able to receive and transmit information from this universal energy field.

One potential mechanism for this connection is through the pineal gland's role in producing melatonin. Melatonin is a hormone that regulates sleep-wake cycles and has also been shown to have antioxidant properties. Some researchers believe that melatonin may also play a role in facilitating communication with the collective consciousness.

The Evidence for and Against the Collective Consciousness Theory

There is no definitive scientific evidence to support the existence of a collective consciousness. However, there are some anecdotal reports and personal experiences that suggest a connection between individuals and a universal energy field.

Some proponents of the collective consciousness theory argue that the synchronicity of events, such as coincidences and shared experiences, is evidence of a deeper connection between all living beings. Others point to the phenomenon of group consciousness, where large groups of people seem to be connected by a shared energy field.

Critics of the collective consciousness theory argue that these phenomena can be explained by other factors, such as chance, coincidence, or shared cultural beliefs. They also point out that there is no scientific evidence to support the existence of a universal energy field.

The Implications of Collective Consciousness

If the collective consciousness exists, it could have profound implications for our understanding of human consciousness and our place in the universe. It could suggest that we are all interconnected at a deeper level, sharing thoughts, emotions, and experiences. This could have implications for social, political, and environmental issues, as it suggests that our actions can have a ripple effect on the entire planet.

Conclusion

The concept of collective consciousness is a fascinating and controversial one. While there is no definitive scientific evidence to support its existence, it is a topic that continues to intrigue researchers and spiritual seekers alike. The pineal gland, with its unique role in human consciousness and its potential connection to higher states of awareness, may offer insights into the nature of collective consciousness. As our understanding of the pineal gland and the human mind continues to evolve, we may gain a deeper appreciation for the interconnectedness of all things.

Chapter 23: The Pineal Gland and the Future of Human Consciousness

Introduction

The pineal gland, a small, pea-sized structure located deep within the brain, has long been associated with spiritual enlightenment and higher consciousness. As our understanding of the pineal gland continues to evolve, so too does our appreciation for its potential role in shaping the future of human consciousness. In this chapter, we will explore the implications of pineal gland activation for the future of humanity, examining the potential benefits and challenges that may arise.

The Potential Benefits of Pineal Gland Activation

The activation of the pineal gland is believed to have the potential to unlock new levels of consciousness and human potential. Some of the potential benefits of pineal gland activation include:

- **Enhanced spiritual awareness:** The pineal gland may serve as a gateway to higher consciousness, allowing us to connect with a universal energy field and gain access to spiritual knowledge and wisdom.
- **Increased creativity and problem-solving abilities:** The pineal gland may be involved in creative thinking and problem-solving, and its activation could enhance these abilities.
- **Improved mental and emotional health:** The pineal gland plays a role in regulating mood and emotions. Activating the pineal gland may help to improve mental and emotional well-being.
- **Enhanced intuition and psychic abilities:** Some people believe that the pineal gland is associated with intuition and psychic abilities. Activating the pineal gland may enhance these abilities.

The Potential Challenges of Pineal Gland Activation

While the potential benefits of pineal gland activation are significant, there are also potential challenges to consider. These challenges may include:

- **Unintended side effects:** Some practices or substances used to activate the pineal gland may have unintended side effects, such as hallucinations, anxiety, or changes in mood.
- **Ethical dilemmas:** The pursuit of spiritual enlightenment and higher consciousness can raise ethical questions, particularly when it involves the use of substances or practices that may be harmful or addictive.
- **Social implications:** The activation of the pineal gland may lead to changes in social behavior and relationships, which could have both positive and negative consequences.

The Future of Pineal Gland Research

As research into the pineal gland continues to advance, we can expect to learn more about its role in human consciousness and behavior. New technologies and scientific techniques may provide us with deeper insights into the pineal gland's functions and its potential for activation.

It is also possible that future research will develop new methods for safely and effectively activating the pineal gland. These methods may involve the use of specific substances, meditation techniques, or other interventions.

Conclusion

The pineal gland is a fascinating organ with the potential to unlock new levels of human consciousness. While there are challenges and risks associated with pineal gland activation, the potential benefits are significant. As research continues to advance, we can expect to learn more about the pineal gland's role in our lives and its potential to shape the future of humanity.

Chapter 24: The Pineal Gland and the Collective Consciousness

Introduction

The pineal gland, a small, pea-sized structure located deep within the brain, has long been associated with spiritual enlightenment and higher consciousness. In recent years, there has been growing interest in the idea that the pineal gland may play a role in connecting us to a collective consciousness, a universal energy field that unites all living beings. In this chapter, we will explore the concept of collective consciousness and its potential relationship to the pineal gland.

Collective Consciousness: A Definition

Collective consciousness, also known as the global consciousness or the noosphere, is a hypothetical field of energy that connects all living beings. Proponents of this theory argue that we are all interconnected at a deeper level, sharing thoughts, emotions, and experiences.

The concept of collective consciousness has been explored by various philosophers, scientists, and spiritual leaders. Carl Jung, for example, believed that the collective consciousness was a shared pool of archetypal images and symbols that influence our thoughts and behaviors.

The Pineal Gland and Collective Consciousness

Some researchers believe that the pineal gland may play a role in connecting us to the collective consciousness. They argue that the pineal gland may be able to receive and transmit information from this universal energy field.

One potential mechanism for this connection is through the pineal gland's role in producing melatonin. Melatonin is a hormone that regulates sleep-wake cycles and has also been shown to have antioxidant properties. Some researchers believe that melatonin may also play a role in facilitating communication with the collective consciousness.

The Evidence for and Against the Collective Consciousness Theory

There is no definitive scientific evidence to support the existence of a collective consciousness. However, there are some anecdotal reports and personal experiences that suggest a connection between individuals and a universal energy field.

Some proponents of the collective consciousness theory argue that the synchronicity of events, such as coincidences and shared experiences, is evidence of a deeper connection between all living beings. Others point to the phenomenon of group consciousness, where large groups of people seem to be connected by a shared energy field.

Critics of the collective consciousness theory argue that these phenomena can be explained by other factors, such as chance, coincidence, or shared cultural beliefs. They also point out that there is no scientific evidence to support the existence of a universal energy field.

The Implications of Collective Consciousness

If the collective consciousness exists, it could have profound implications for our understanding of human consciousness and our place in the universe. It could suggest that we are all interconnected at a deeper level, sharing thoughts, emotions, and experiences. This could have implications for social, political, and environmental issues, as it suggests that our actions can have a ripple effect on the entire planet.

Conclusion

The concept of collective consciousness is a fascinating and controversial one. While there is no definitive scientific evidence to support its existence, it is a topic that continues to intrigue researchers and spiritual seekers alike. The pineal gland, with its unique role in human consciousness and its potential connection to higher states of awareness, may offer insights into the nature of collective consciousness. As our understanding of the pineal gland and the human mind continues to evolve, we may gain a deeper appreciation for the interconnectedness of all things.

Chapter 25: The Future of Pineal Gland Research

Introduction

The pineal gland, a small, pea-sized structure located deep within the brain, has long been a subject of fascination and speculation. As our understanding of the pineal gland continues to evolve, so too does our appreciation for its potential role in human consciousness and well-being. In this final chapter, we will explore the future of pineal gland research, examining the potential directions that this field may take in the coming years.

Emerging Technologies and Research Methods

Advances in technology are providing researchers with new tools to study the pineal gland and its functions. Some of the emerging technologies that may play a significant role in future research include:

- **Brain imaging techniques:** Techniques such as magnetic resonance imaging (MRI) and positron emission tomography (PET) can be used to study the structure and function of the pineal gland in living humans.
- **Genetic analysis:** Genetic analysis can help to identify the genes involved in pineal gland development and function.
- **Nanotechnology:** Nanotechnology may be used to develop new methods for studying and manipulating the pineal gland at the cellular level.

Potential Directions for Future Research

In addition to these technological advancements, there are several areas of research that may be fruitful in the coming years. These include:

- **The pineal gland and aging:** Further research is needed to understand how the pineal gland changes with age and the potential consequences of these changes.
- **The pineal gland and neurodegenerative diseases:** The pineal gland may play a role in neurodegenerative diseases such as Alzheimer's disease and Parkinson's disease. Future research may explore the potential for targeting the pineal gland to develop new treatments for these conditions.
- **The pineal gland and mental health:** The pineal gland's role in regulating mood and emotions suggests that it may be involved in mental health disorders such as depression and anxiety. Future research may explore the potential for targeting the pineal gland to develop new treatments for these conditions.
- **The pineal gland and consciousness:** The relationship between the pineal gland and human consciousness remains a fascinating area of research. Future studies may explore the potential for the pineal gland to facilitate communication with higher consciousness or other dimensions of reality.

Ethical Considerations

As research into the pineal gland continues to advance, it is important to consider the ethical implications of this work. Researchers must ensure that their studies are conducted ethically and that the well-being of participants is protected. It is also important to be mindful of the potential social and cultural implications of research into the pineal gland.

Conclusion

The pineal gland is a complex and fascinating organ with the potential to unlock new levels of human consciousness and well-being. As research continues to advance, we can expect to learn more about its functions and its role in shaping our lives. By understanding the pineal gland and its potential, we can take steps to optimize its function and embrace the extraordinary possibilities that it offers.

www.ingramcontent.com/pod-product-compliance
Lightning Source LLC
Chambersburg PA
CBHW062104220526
45471CB00010B/3599